A Psychoanalytic Understanding of Trauma

A Psychoanalytic Understanding of Trauma presents a theory of the nature of trauma and post-traumatic mental functioning based on the concept of the 'zero process'.

Joseph Fernando presents a novel, comprehensive, and clinically useful theory of trauma. The author first presents theories of trauma and describes the zero process, related to the breakdown of various ego functions, such as memory and integration, during trauma. Rather than replacing Freud's ideas of the primary process and repression, Fernando expands on the idea of the mind to include both types of functioning, identifies how they can be differentiated, and examines the different therapeutic techniques they require. He also considers how trauma impacts the construction of reality, the role of human development, the relation of trauma and borderline disorders, and the development of therapeutic technique. Through the unique illustration and narration of cases of three patients, Fernando presents conceptual and clinical innovations.

A Psychoanalytic Understanding of Trauma will be of great interest to psychoanalysts and psychoanalytic psychotherapists in practice and in training.

Joseph Fernando is the director of the Toronto Institute of Psychoanalysis, Canada. He has had a full-time psychoanalytic clinical practice, and taught and supervised students, for over 30 years. He is a Gradiva award winning author and has published widely and presented his ideas internationally.

Psychoanalytic Ideas and Applications Series
Series Editor: Silvia Flechner

IPA Publications Committee
Fred Busch, Natacha Delgado, Nergis Güleç, Thomas Marcacci, Carlos Moguillansky, Rafael Mondrzak, Angela M. Vuotto, Gabriela Legoretta (consultant)

"Dr. Fernando is an exciting psychoanalytic thinker and contemporary ego psychologist, whose creativity, riveting clinical acumen and scholarship show especially in the presentation of his new concept, "zero process" in illumination of how a traumatized person's mind functions. This work is fresh and brilliantly helpful to everyday practice."
  – **Rosemary Balsam M.D.**, *Yale Medical School; Western New England Institute for Psychoanalysis*

"With a deft blending of the modern conflict theory of psychoanalysis with advanced studies of psychic trauma, the perspective of drives, and the work of Bion and contemporary French contributors, Joseph Fernando offers us an expanded and deepened view of the traumatized mind. An original contribution in this setting is his concept of the "zero process" denoting the mental functioning left over after the ordinary construction of reality is shattered. Providing ample clinical illustrations, he lucidly presents the explicatory and therapeutic value of such conceptualization. This is an important book and deserves our serious attention."
  – **Salman Akhtar, M.D.** *Professor of Psychiatry, Jefferson Medical College Training and Supervising Analyst, Psychoanalytic Center of Philadelphia*

"With his zero process theory, Joseph Fernando develops a unique psychoanalytic theory of trauma based on Freud's concepts and theories. With his theoretical approach and his detailed clinical descriptions of post-traumatic memories, symptoms, and disorders, he opens up a deeper understanding of how the traumatic mind works. He succeeds in shedding new light on hitherto inadequately understood traumatic phenomena, thus providing new directions for their therapeutic treatment. Fernando's book is an outstanding theoretical and clinically convincing contribution to the field of trauma research."
  – **Werner Bohleber, PhD,** *Psychoanalyst, Former Editor of the German Psychoanalytic Journal PSYCHE*

"There are many ideas in this new book that I totally subscribe to; others that, unsurprisingly, I would formulate differently. What really matters, however, is that the ideas contained here are at once bold, rational, thought-provoking, and clinically useful. Joseph Fernando's work in general, and this book in particular, demonstrate something of great importance to me: that metapsychology is alive and kicking; that it is a field open to revision and to new and original contributions; that it is inseparable from – and vital for – clinical thinking in psychoanalysis."
  – **Dominique Scarfone,** *Training and supervising analyst at the Canadian Psychoanalytic Society and Institute*

A Psychoanalytic Understanding of Trauma

Post-Traumatic Mental Functioning, the Zero Process, and the Construction of Reality

Joseph Fernando

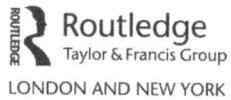
Routledge
Taylor & Francis Group

LONDON AND NEW YORK

Cover image: Getty

First published 2023
by Routledge
4 Park Square, Milton Park, Abingdon, Oxon OX14 4RN

and by Routledge
605 Third Avenue, New York, NY 10158

Routledge is an imprint of the Taylor & Francis Group, an informa business

© 2023 Joseph Fernando

British Library Cataloguing-in-Publication Data
A catalogue record for this book is available from the British Library

ISBN: 978-1-032-25443-2 (hbk)
ISBN: 978-1-032-25442-5 (pbk)
ISBN: 978-1-003-28321-8 (ebk)

DOI: 10.4324/9781003283218

Typeset in Palatino
by MPS Limited, Dehradun

Contents

Series Editor's Foreword

The Publications Committee of the International Psychoanalytic Association continues, with the present volume, the series "Psychoanalytic Ideas and Applications."

The aim of this series is to focus on the scientific output of significant authors whose works are outstanding contributions to the development of the psychoanalytic field and to set out relevant ideas and themes, generated during the history of psychoanalysis, which deserve to be known and discussed by present-day psychoanalysts.

The relationship between psychoanalytic ideas and their applications needs to be put forward from the perspective of theory, clinical practice, and research, to maintain their validity for contemporary psychoanalysis.

The Publication's Committee's objective is to share these ideas with the psychoanalytic community and with professionals in other related disciplines, to expand their knowledge and generate a productive exchange between the text and the reader. The IPA Publications Committee is pleased to publish the book *A Psychoanalytic Understanding of Trauma* by Joseph Fernando. Dr. Joseph Fernando is a training and supervising analyst at the Toronto Institute of Psychoanalysis; he has extensive clinical and teaching experience over many years and has published widely.

Dr. Fernando is a most interesting and creative psychoanalytic thinker. In this book, he skillfully describes the way in which mental functioning is deeply affected when the healthy process of construction of reality is devastated by traumatic events. His thought-provoking concept of "zero process" sheds light on our understanding of the way in which a traumatized mind functions. The zero process is discussed in its relation to time, in relation to the type of memory associated with it, in its connection to the process of symbolization, and the construction of reality. The present volume is an outgrowth of his previous book "The Processes of Defense" which won the 2010 Gradiva prize for psychoanalytic theory. In the Introduction to the current book, Dr. Fernando summarizes his theoretical path from his first book to the theory of the zero process. The author extends the theory of trauma and zero process, both developing it in more detail and broadening its scope. He examines in more depth the nature of the disruption of certain ego functions, such as memory and integration, during the traumatic process. In this manner, his theory of trauma has become both more nuanced and more radical than his previous formulations regarding the nature of post-traumatic psychic functioning.

The originality of the author's contribution lies in his ability to bring together Freud's theory emphasizing the ego psychology theory of conflict, including the drive theory, with the work of important contemporary analysts from different psychoanalytic cultures such as Bion, Botella, Scarfone, and Roussillon to name a few.

Not only does the author offer an elaborated and expanded theoretical view of the effect of trauma, he also provides three extensive clinical cases that bring the theory to life by illustrating the way in which his theoretical perspective can be used in clinical situations.

The book is skillfully organized in five chapters. After an introductory chapter, Dr. Fernando takes up the question of our understanding of the mind and how it is affected by trauma. Here is where Dr. Fernando's original contributions are introduced, including the idea of the zero process, which is responsible for the freezing of elements of the traumatic moment. He also considers specific forms of zero process defenses, zero process structures such as introjects and zero process drives. Other chapters deal with the question of the construction of reality, the relation of trauma to borderline disorders, and therapeutic technique.

We are thankful to Dr. Fernando for having provided an exciting addition to the understanding of traumatic phenomena and for providing new ways of conceptualizing the working of the mind in these states as well as providing us with new clinical directions. Dr. Fernando's book is an outstanding theoretical and clinical contribution to the field of trauma.

It will without doubt be of interest to the psychoanalytic community as well as to anyone interested in the field of trauma.

Gabriela Legorreta
Series Editor
Chair, IPA Publications Committee

Preface

The reader will notice as they make their way through this book that there are numerous references to the ideas developed in my previous book, on the processes of defense. They will also notice that at some points I reference my next book, on development, the superego, and sociohistorical issues. While they did not start out this way, this series of books have acquired something of a sequence and a structure. This book and the last one explore basic psychoanalytic concepts and their clinical correlates, in order to reformulate many established concepts such as denial and repression, and propose some new ones, such as compound defenses, temporal shifting, and the zero process. From these a theory of forms of mental functioning, and of forms of mental dynamics that are built on them, emerges. The third book, to follow, will use these ideas and this theory, in pushing towards a new and deeper understanding of the development and functioning of those most human of phenomena: internal objects, morality, and the superego. From there, a deeper exploration of socio-historical, and very much present day, issues such as societal regression, as well as the evolution of the human mind, beckon.

These explorations, reformulations, and innovations have been achieved using the psychoanalytic investigational method, and a basic ego psychological conceptual framework. This framework is most useful not as a settled theory, but rather as a way of approaching the mind as a collection of very many independent, even if interacting and intertwined, capacities, functions, and tendencies. Each of these enters into complex causal networks as an independent factor, not reducible to any others. For instance trauma cannot be reduced to conflict, or to relational issues, nor can these two, or others, be reduced to the effects of trauma. I hope this point of view, stated here in very condensed and austere form, will gain content and meaning through the extended discussions, and detailed stories from patients, that follow.

Joseph Fernando

Acknowledgements

My ideas on trauma have developed in the context of, and as a consequence of, discussions with many colleagues, students, and patients. My friend Jim Deutsch invited me to present at the Toronto chapter of the International Neuropsychoanalysis Society that he headed – which is where one of the participants suggested the term "zero process" for the still germinating ideas about post-traumatic functioning that I described. I discussed with Cyril Levitt the ideas in my first book, including the zero process. After the publication of that book I spent a number of years researching in preparation for a work on what I have come to think of as "Evolutionary Psychoanalysis." Cyril suggested, when I asked him what he thought, that it might be better to take a break from this rather vast research project, to concentrate on something more manageable and doable. And thus the work on this book began.

Charles Levin, editor of the Canadian Journal of Psychoanalysis at the time, was very energetic in his support of my first book, reviewing it and organizing, through the Journal, a one day conference on the book in Toronto, the discussions of which the Journal published. Werner Bohleber kindly agreed to come from Germany to headline that conference. He presented a very thoughtful discussion and detailed critiques of my ideas, which were stimulating to me. As editor of the leading German language journal, *Psyche*, he helped in the publication of my paper on trauma and the zero process in German. He and his wife Marianne Leuzinger-Bohleber are two of the foremost, and most thoughtful, international investigators of trauma, and I have benefited from their ideas, from mutual discussions, and from their lively and warm company during meals in New York, Prague, and Mexico City. Eva Papiasvili, at that time the North American co-chair of the IPA Encyclopaedic dictionary (IRED), asked me to contribute something on the zero process to a number of entries of this important project, which led to my greater involvement with IRED as Eva moved up to chair the entire endeavour. She has been from the start extremely positive and supportive of my work and its dissemination.

I met Tony Kris in 1993 at the Amsterdam IPA Congress, and from that time forward he was supportive of me and my work as only Tony could be. Steve Ablon, whom I met sometime after that in London at the Anna Freud Centre, invited me as a discussant at the Boston Psychoanalytic Society. Steve and Tony then got together and invited me to be a member of their discussion group at the Centre for Advanced Psychoanalytic Studies (CAPS) at Princeton. CAPS group 2 has provided a wonderful atmosphere for lively discussion of ideas during our meetings, walks, and while eating and imbibing various wines and spirits. The group has included, during the 10 years of my membership, Tony Kris (who sadly passed away last year), Steve Ablon, Richard Honig, Rosemary Balsam, Larry Levenson, Dwarakanath (Dwarky) Rao, Helène Keable, Barry Landau, Nancy Chodorow, Alexandra Harrison, Jon Meyer, Lisa Buchberg, Melvin Lansky, Karen Gilmore, Stacey Fry, and Elizabeth Wilson.

My friend Sarah Usher, and her husband, and fellow Toronto Maple Leafs fan, Gary McKay, have provided much encouragement and many laughs. Sarah is always one book ahead of me on the publication trail, which keeps me soldiering on.

These are just a few of the many colleagues who have encouraged me, challenged me, and influenced me, in my development as a psychoanalytic clinician and theoretician. My editor has informed me of length limits on this book, so I am forced to stop here (as they do when the music plays at the awards ceremonies), and just mention as a group all of my colleagues at the Toronto Psychoanalytic Society and Institute, in other parts of Canada, and internationally. We may argue and challenge each other, but we are one large family underneath all that.

And speaking of family, I come finally to my wife Susan and children Wren, Nicky, Kiri, and Jonathan. They have been genuinely encouraging of, and excited for, me and full of interesting ideas and questions about the work. Wren chose the cover photo and, as our resident artist, would have drawn an even better one if only I'd thought to ask her in time – next book. My mother, who has herself published extensively in her field of parasitology, was interested in my progress, and my sister Shanti, a political scientist who also has published quite a bit, had excellent advice on many aspects of writing and publishing.

Introduction

Given its presence in both the professional and public domains, trauma seems to be an idea whose time has arrived. It is, however, an idea whose time had arrived many times previously. One major arrival occurred in the later half of the 19th century, with the dawn of medical psychology. Pierre Janet (1920) and Joseph Breuer and Sigmund Freud (1895) are the best known of a number of investigators who asserted both the traumatic aetiology of hysteria and the psychological (rather than physical) understanding of disorders that followed upon accidents, such as "railway spine". Trauma is hard to hold onto, and is slippery in more ways than one, so that what we learn about it is often forgotten. In order to understand how and why trauma has these characteristics, I invite you to join me on a journey.

The journey will be to a new world, though not an unexplored one, as the continent of trauma has certainly not only been discovered but its landscape explored and mapped out. I hope to demonstrate in the pages that follow that there is still more to explore—that we can go deeper into this land. However, one of the main themes of this book is that in order to explore further, we need also to look more closely at the maps we have been using to navigate and understand this continent of the mind. These maps are the concepts that we use to understand trauma and post-traumatic problems. I will be contending that many of our maps, both old and new, contain crucial errors—errors which have led us astray in our explorations. The landscape of trauma and post-traumatic mental functioning is a strange place. A place where time stands still much of the time, then goes forward at breakneck speed for a bit, and then rewinds to the beginning, returning to its former frozen state. A place where specific parts, such as an image or a feeling, do not connect with each other, but instead loom large and ominous at times as we travel by them, only to disappear as quickly as they appeared. In our maps this world, so different from our everyday experience, has been confused with other strange lands. As explorers discovered the land of trauma, they mistook

DOI: 10.4324/9781003283218-1

it for other far-off lands that they had heard of, just as European explorers felt they had discovered India or other parts of Asia when they came upon the Americas. The way the mind functions after trauma has been thought to be the same as the functioning of the early infantile mind, or it has been conflated with disorders in which the inner world of feelings and drives cannot be modulated and contained, such as borderline and psychotic conditions.

One of the guiding ideas in this book is that by more clearly understanding what trauma is not, we will more deeply understand what it is. If we extend the idea of trauma so that all sorts of impingements are trauma, and all sorts of, perhaps even all, mental disturbances are thought to be caused by trauma, then it becomes hard to see what trauma really is. It becomes too diffuse and hard to bring into focus. At the same time, this extension of the concept leads to a loss of valuable and hard-won insights into other continents of the mind.

After describing some of the basic aspects of trauma in the first chapter, I will in the second introduce the concept of the zero process as the form of mental functioning left over after the breakdown during trauma of the regular, everyday construction of reality. The idea that there is such a form of post-traumatic mental functioning is not a new one, as many people have made such a proposal, and given this form of functioning different names. I will point out the similarities between the zero process and the ideas of other authors. By exploring more deeply different aspects of trauma and post-traumatic functioning, which are the subjects of chapter two, differences will also become evident. The key more general difference is that I have fashioned the concept of the zero process so as not to replace other ideas, such as Freud's differentiation between the primary process (a mode of functioning related to drives and affects which reigns in the deeper unconscious) and the secondary process (the more rational, reality-oriented form of functioning used by our ego). Rather than replacement, I am proposing differentiation and addition. I delineate specific characteristics of post-traumatic functioning which differentiate it from other forms of mental functioning. To give an example, both the zero process of trauma and the primary process related to the deeper emotional mind can be described as not having the usual time sense of the more reality-oriented secondary process. But they are timeless—outside of time—in very different ways. Post-traumatic states involve something like the freezing of a present moment or sets of moments, so that they live on as a perpetual present. There is often some ordering of these moments, and they can be triggered and relived in displaced and distorted form in a sequence, or they can be projected into the future. But the differentiation of past, present, and future, the abstraction and integration of these, and the effects of change over time, are all missing in the zero process. In the primary process there is much more movement and interaction of elements and affects, as they fuse with each other, or displace their energy onto other objects or onto objects in the outer world. But time does not effect the wishes and memories in this deeper, emotional part of the mind, which remain as fresh as the day they were formed. I have briefly touched on these differences, which will be elaborated on later, to demonstrate the sorts of distinctions upon which the idea of the zero process is based.

An important idea in psychoanalytic literature, which attempts to understand the differences between Freud's primary process and post-traumatic phenomena, is that of trauma and unrepresented states. These enigmatic states have been explored by many authors, and especially in the French (Rousillon, 2011; Botella, 2014) psychoanalytic tradition. This area of inquiry is quite diverse, as an example growing in France out of the investigation of psychosomatic disorders, which seem to involve early disturbances in the capacity to symbolize (Marty, 1968; De M'Uzan, 2003). Freud's concept of deferred action, in which something that was not understood at the time of its occurrence has an effect at a later date, such as the Wolf Man's witnessing of the primal scene (Freud, 1918), has also been connected to trauma and lack of proper representation when the trauma first occurs. Here too it has been especially French authors who have taken to the use of this idea of "après coup" in conceptualizing their material. A good introduction to the range of ideas on unrepresented states is the collection of papers edited by Levine et al. (2013). I will discuss the literature related to theories of unrepresented states in a number of places in chapters two and three (sections "A Trip Down Memory Lane" and "Zero Process Denial and Temporal Shifting").

Along with its effect on symbolization and representation, and as a consequence of these effects, trauma also bends and distorts time. Temporality is a common topic among trauma theorists, for instance with the idea of après coup used by Lacanian and other French workers, and the important work of Dominique Scarfone (2006, 2014, 2015) on the "actual unconscious" and its relation to the "unpast." I will attempt to show how detailed inquiry into the nature and dynamics of the zero process allows us to understand some of the deeper underlying dynamics of these temporal distortions. These dynamics are discussed especially in the section in chapter three, "Zero Process Denial and Temporal Shifting," but are a theme throughout this book.

What I see myself doing is not so much presenting a completely new theory in opposition to other theories of trauma, but rather as trying to untie a set of knots, in which single concepts have been applied to disparate phenomena. The phenomena that we actually observe contain a mixture of various forms of functioning such as the primary process, the secondary process, and the zero process, as well as being influenced by persistent aspects of very early life, various developmental interferences, and constitutional abilities and deficits. Concepts such as the zero process, as well as Freud's idea of the primary process, sit at some distance from these observed phenomena. But by making certain crucial distinctions, these concepts allow us to sort out these phenomena and disentangle the various mental states and dynamics involved in a way that allows deeper insight, and is clinically helpful. The demonstration that this is in fact so is the work of this book.

I have been inspired by the various authors mentioned and others, to fashion concepts specific to trauma. One of the most influential psychoanalysts who proposed a new set of concepts for different mental states was Wilfred Bion (1962), who suggested that the raw input from experience, which he called beta elements, needed to be subject to the alpha function (usually provided by the caregiver in early infancy) to be transformed into our more regular experience. From Bion I got the idea of the need for a separate concept to denote the radically concrete, unsymbolized, and unintegrated bits and pieces nature of post-traumatic memories. Also, his work suggests that this bits and pieces form of mental reality is not merely a product of trauma, but in fact that all experience starts like this and needs a set of profound transformations (the alpha function) to become what we take to be regular experience. Trauma interferes with these transformations. However, it will become clear from the ensuing discussions that the main feature distinguishing Bion's theory from my own is that Bion traces the difficulties of the retention of beta elements to failures in the caretaker's alpha function in early childhood. In other words he connects, and at times perhaps he, and certainly many who use his theories, conflate, the traumatic process and the developmental processes, by using the same set of concepts for both. My own view is that while there are many connections between these two, they are at their base distinct processes with differentiable causes and dynamics. It is especially in chapter four, on understanding borderline disorders, and in the discussions of therapeutic techniques in chapter five, that these distinctions will be shown to be useful.

The distinctions I make in this book are an extension of a project that began with my work on defenses (Fernando, 2009). In that book I distinguished between the effects of overwhelming from internal sources such as drives and strong affects, and overwhelming from outside. I described the very different forms of defense used against external as compared to internal phenomena. This led me also to note that at the clinical observational level, the dynamics and outcomes of overwhelming from the internal sources are quite different from those that come from the external overwhelming that we know as trauma. And this led to the beginnings of a description of zero process theory. Having laid the groundwork for these basic distinctions in my previous work, I will in this book be taking zero process theory deeper and further: deeper into a more detailed description of its formation and characteristics, and further in seeing what zero process memory fragments get up to once they are set free into the wider world.

The first part of this endeavour, the deeper exploration of the nature of trauma and the zero process, will be undertaken in the first two chapters. Each of these chapters begins by jumping straight into a clinical case and the details of a patient's experience of serious trauma. These provide clinical and experiential grounding for the conceptual expositions, relating to the nature of the traumatic process, of zero process traumatic memories, and of memories more generally. The last three chapters explore some key applications of the theory of the zero process. In chapter three we will see that many things, such as drives and defenses, can have a zero process version, and that the nature of the zero process can help us explain many enigmatic phenomena, such as those inner entities, including our superego, which seem so real and separate from us, even as they live inside us, and the extreme version of this—dissociative identity disorder (DID – formerly called multiple personality disorder). Chapter four takes a deep dive into the dynamics and causation of borderline personality disorder. This disorder has been claimed by many investigators to be caused by trauma, more specifically by a certain type of early relational trauma referred to as developmental trauma. This chapter will give us a chance to discuss in more depth the relation between trauma and development, as well as delving further into another theme of this book—the relationship between the zero process and the primary process. Discussing each of these topics in relation to a specific clinical problem will demonstrate the clinical usefulness of these theoretical ideas. The final chapter will continue this demonstration more directly, by surveying the field of trauma therapy. We will see that a clear understanding of the nature of the zero process allows us to understand how the many different forms of trauma therapy work, as well as helping us to fashion new forms of intervention.

I compared the discovery and exploration of trauma to the discovery and exploration of the Americas by Europeans. But of course when these explorers arrived there were already people there who had lived in and travelled through the land for many thousands of years. Just so with trauma—people have lived in this strange land since the birth of the human species. In fact the land of trauma, just as the land discovered by European explorers, predates our species. We all dwell in this continent to some extent, although often with little awareness that this is the case. While my summary of this book so far may have made it seem that it involves largely theoretical discussions, it is in fact filled with stories from people who have dwelt in the land of trauma longer, and more deeply, than most. They have generously allowed me to tell their stories here, so that we may all come to understand something further about the true nature of this land, and thus better aid those who have lost their way in it.

(After the Conclusion there is a Glossary of the new terms that are introduced and used in this book. I would urge the reader to familiarize themselves with these by referring to them when the terms occur in the book. At their first occurrence after this introduction, they are indicated in **bold** letters.)

Chapter 1

The Traumatic Process

A young girl is at the dinner table with her father and two siblings. She is only four and a half. The two siblings are younger. She has had a very busy young life. Two siblings were born, who took her mother's attention away. At about age three, she developed croup, and was kept in a tent in hospital. She remembers breaking out of it and wandering the hospital corridor till a nurse found her. When her mother was pregnant with the youngest, cancer was discovered. She was treated, but over the next year and a half she deteriorated and finally ended up in hospital, thin and wasting away. The young girl visited her there. She remembers lying beside her mother on the hospital bed. This day at dinner her father, with the youngest on his lap, tells the children that their mother is not going to be coming home. He says that they will have to stick together as a family. As he says this the young girl has a powerful physical feeling, that she has been punched in the stomach. She cannot breathe or eat. And a darkness, experienced not symbolically but actually, as darkness, enters into her through her belly.

This young girl eventually, as an adult, came to see me for help with her feeling that she was unsure about her relationship, and for certain anxieties. She told me about what had happened to her mother. She felt this may have had something to do with her difficulties, and had made some connections between this past event and her present difficulties. There is much to be said about the events both before and after this pivotal moment, and we will get a chance to visit some of these later but for now, I would like to concentrate on the moment itself. My patient, Cordelia, did not go very far into the details of the incident when she would mention it, but would merely recount what her father had said and how bad she had felt. The incident was not repressed, but rather Cordelia avoided thinking of it. The details I have mentioned only emerged with repeated retelling. In some instances of trauma, the avoidance can be almost total, but in her case it seemed to be directed mainly at going into too much detail, at the emotional intensity, and at the connections of the incident to other things. One connection she did make right from the start was that each of

DOI: 10.4324/9781003283218-2

her long-term relationships had lasted about four years, at which time she felt a powerful need to leave.

Cordelia was in psychotherapy, twice a week for most of the time, sitting up. Later she began a four times weekly psychoanalysis. Let's look at a few sessions a couple of years into her therapy: she comes into a session and starts talking of how she is quite angry at her husband for not doing various things she thinks he should, to take care of his recovery from a serious illness he has had. She is not a pushy person in general, she says (and her behaviour in therapy bears this out), but she is pushy in relation to people's health (she has in fact made health recommendations to me as well.) People were never doing enough, and she would get angry at them for resisting her advice. She remembers this going on at least from the age of 20, when she began pushing remedies on her somewhat reluctant father. I say something about whether there is some pleasure as she does this. "It doesn't feel good when I'm doing it," Cordelia says with some feeling, and a look that shows distaste or even disgust. "I get a funny feeling in my stomach when I think of doing it. Like with my mother." (We both know she is referring to the incident when she was told about her mother's death.)

"If you stick with that feeling, what else comes up?"

"It's like a black hole in my stomach, that would suck everything into it." She visibly shudders as she describes this. "It feels like death itself. But maybe it's my aggression as well. I think of my fear of intruders. They seem like that same black hole—but maybe they are really my own aggression."

"Come back to haunt you, and attack you."

"It really does seem like it. I think of the dream of the murderer, at night. (A dream dreamt at the start of therapy, of a murderer killing people and burying them at night, while the patient, in fear, watched and tried to hide.) Was it me?" Cordelia becomes somewhat overwhelmed, looking shaken. It is the end of the session, and I ask if she is OK to leave. She says she will be fine, but she is a bit surprised by the strength of the feelings.

At the next session, the next week, Cordelia returns to the need to save people. "I pushed [her step mother] to give my father some different remedies for his health problems. She said he was OK. I was about to push some more, but then I held myself back. I tried to let it go. I didn't say anything more, but it was hard."

She then brings up the incident when she was told of her mother's death. She repeats what was said by her father, which she had described previously, that they had to stick together as a family. "I lost my appetite. I may have had food in my mouth, but I don't think I could eat any more. It's like I could not swallow, like my food was dry. Time stopped. It was like a black hole. It was like I died, in that moment. For that moment.

A frozen moment with a black hole. Like the intruder in the house; it's dark like the night when the intruder comes in. Is the intruder maybe death itself?"

There is a silence, and I say, "it all went inside you."

"Maybe if I kept it inside me, I could stop time."

"And save your mother."

Cordelia is crying through the last part of this exchange and says, as she has tears in her eyes, that she is not sure why the tears are coming now. She would often start to cry, even at earlier times when we had talked about that fateful night. This may seem unsurprising, to cry as one talked of hearing of the death of one's mother. But the crying would come somewhat unbidden and often surprise Cordelia. It seemed at times to descend upon her, rather than grow out of an integrated retelling of a story. It could gain in intensity quite suddenly, but also disappear quickly.

In the next four sessions, Cordelia has dreams and experiences, all of which lead back to the element of surprise. She dreams that she is living with a past boyfriend. They were together and it seemed really solid. But then he calls her and says, "instead of being here for dinner, why don't you just stop by for lunch?" Cordelia goes downstairs to tell her father and stepmother, and sees coffee on the wall, making a mess. It is devastating for Cordelia, this going from one extreme to the other. She thought the relationship was solid and serious, and all of a sudden it isn't. I connect this to unexpectedly hearing of her mother's death. She notes that she left this boyfriend four years into the relationship. She had felt an urgent need to get out of the relationship, as if she were trapped and would die in it. But soon after she, to the surprise of her boyfriend, announced that she was leaving, she herself felt bereft, alone and desperate to get back to him. But as she went back and forth like this, unsure, her boyfriend moved on. Later in the session we discuss adolescence, where longing for her mother and father reappeared, as did her anger, enacted with her stepmother especially. "All I wanted was love." A dream in the next session is quite startling: "I was standing there. An attack dog hits the ground, like it was falling from the sky. It's a pit bull type of attack dog that runs at me, and I take a breath in, a gasp, and wake up. I was scared. It was the gasp I really remember, as the dog jumped at me." She wondered about her own aggression—if this was the dog. The gasp reminds her of when she was told of her mother's death, a punch in the stomach. She has just heard of a pit bull attack in which the dog had come from the neighbour's back yard and had killed a woman in her own back yard. Later in the session, there are memories of her mother with her back turned to her, and examples of how angry Cordelia can get when she is not listened to.

Lack of Preparedness and Being Overwhelmed

One specific characteristic that appeared again and again in relation to Cordelia being told about her mother's death, was the suddenness of what happened. From the earliest descriptions on, this aspect of trauma has been stressed. Being taken by surprise is not just related to time, however, but also to expectation. And expectation is related to our models, both immediate and more general, of the world. So we could say an event has the possibility of becoming traumatic if it comes on so suddenly and/or is so beyond the regular expectations of the person, that they cannot quickly assimilate it. Of course surprise birthday parties can have these characteristics, but are usually not traumatic. Yet if the surprise party is truly unexpected, if for instance the person has never had one, and never expected to, then they not only will not assimilate the event right away, but may seem in a mild state of shock, and keep repeating, "I can't believe it. I still just can't believe that this is happening." There are characteristics of what we call trauma that can be experienced separately from other aspects. The specific characteristic that the surprise birthday party isolates and demonstrates is the one of not being able to assimilate the incoming sensory input into one's usual model of the world, and the disruption that this can cause.

Cordelia had not been told much about her mother's illness, and certainly had not been told that she was dying. Her father and her mother's parents seem to have been completely overwhelmed by what was happening. It's likely that they were also trying to spare the children upset, as can be seen by their behaviour after the mother's death, of not taking them to the funeral. This is not to say that Cordelia would not have had her suspicions, but they would not have been made explicit in her mind, would have been confused with fantasies, would at times have been pushed aside and denied, and at others assumed frightening proportions. Let's imagine that her father and maternal grandparents had told her, in smaller doses, some of the very upsetting news that they were getting. She would almost certainly have been more overtly upset than she was at hearing the news of her mother's death from her father. She would have been scared, cried, had questions, and had trouble sleeping. What if her mother had told her that she was dying when she visited her in the hospital? It's hard to imagine a more upsetting situation. While the immediate upset would have looked worse, the long-term consequences would almost certainly have been less severe, especially if Cordelia had not only been told these unpleasant truths but been then given emotional support and encouraged to talk about her reactions. But even in a less than ideal version of this, the worst consequences may have been averted.

We might say, when it comes to protecting oneself from being traumatized, that readiness is all. Not every surprise, not every reality which is not part of our expectations, is traumatic. At a slower pace, and in smaller doses, they will lead to some level of emotional upset, but not to trauma. (Certain basic therapeutic techniques are based on this fact.) Emotional upset, even serious emotional upset, is not the same as trauma. In certain respects it is the opposite of trauma. Frustration, upset, and upheaval usually spur adaptation and growth, while trauma brings these to a halt. (Certain modern child-rearing practices that ignore this distinction, treating every potential frustration or upset as a trauma, have extremely bad consequences.) Chronic ongoing upheaval is an intermediate case: it does interfere with development, in some ways similarly to trauma, while at the same time leading to various adaptations. Situations of chronic upheaval usually involve different shock traumas along with ongoing lower level impingements. These have been called type II trauma (Terr, 1995) or strain trauma (Kris, 1956b).

In the latter half of the 1800s, physicians realized that sudden accidents or other shocks seemed to lead to physical symptoms with no obvious physical cause—such as "railway spine" as an aftereffect of train crashes. At first it was thought that these symptoms were caused by physical damage to the brain, but the idea that it was a psychological reaction finally took hold (Micale & Lerner, 2001). Following on these earlier investigations, the two most influential explorers of these reactions, Pierre Janet and Sigmund Freud, developed more sophisticated theories of trauma. The ideas and arguments presented in this book build on the work of these two pioneers. I extend their work in two directions. Firstly, and most straightforwardly, I will delve more deeply into the nature of the processes and dynamics that they so long ago, and others who have followed them more recently, have described. Secondly, I will argue that Janet and Freud, as well as many later influential trauma theorists, at times mixed up very different processes and problems, only one of which is a direct outcome of trauma. This second point is important, I believe, because this mixup of the splitting and psychic instability of borderline dynamics and of various outcomes of developmental interferences with similar seeming, but dynamically and structurally different, post-traumatic phenomena has led to theoretical and clinical problems.

But first, before arguing about what isn't trauma, let's continue to look at what is. Pierre Janet felt that key characteristics of trauma were a product of the failure to assimilate an incident that was too far outside the experiences of the person, and that because of this, actions and feelings that would have been appropriate to the situation were not performed or felt (Van Der Kolk & Van Der Hart, 1995). Symptoms involved versions of the truncated actions and feelings appearing in the present. (We could think of Cordelia trying desperately to "save" any sick person around her, as she could not save her mother.) The theory of trauma and the **zero process** that I will be presenting in the next two chapters begins with Janet's basic understanding of trauma and its aftermath. Because Janet's further development of his theory of the mind, despite many insightful observations, diverges so much from my own, I will not overburden the presentation of my ideas by ongoing comparison with those of Janet or his modern-day followers. (For an excellent exposition of Janet's psychological theories, combining the efforts of many scholars, see Craparo, Ortu, and van der Hart (2019).) I will return to Janet's ideas in chapter five, in discussions of therapeutic technique. In lieu of detailed theoretical comparisons, I present here a quote. In distinguishing post-traumatic hallucinations from those in schizophrenia, Janet notes that hallucinations related to trauma, "imply a problem at the time of the initial event that has not allowed the construction of the story following the laws of memory, which has left the situation unfinished, unsettled, and which caused the need to start it over and over again" (Moskowitz et al., 2019, p. 138, quoting Janet, 1932). This sentence succinctly lays out the basic theory of trauma and the zero process that I will be presenting. As I do this, I will use a psychoanalytic understanding of various ego functions to elucidate further the nature of the traumatic process and of post-traumatic memories, and I will use psychoanalytic dynamic theory to understand what is done to these unprocessed memories—things such as repression, denial, and **zero process defenses** that are specific to trauma.

Breuer and Freud (1895) presented a somewhat similar description of trauma to Janet's, stressing strangulated affects. From this point, Freud took a different fork in the road, going on to emphasize defenses and internal emotional conflicts over external overwhelming and dissociation, developing the methods of free association and interpretation, and making his monumental discoveries of childhood sexuality, the Oedipus complex, transference, repression, and the primary process. One of the reasons I chose Cordelia as a first example is that some of her symptoms are the sort that Janet, Freud, and Breuer first described, and they allow us to comprehend how such symptoms can be investigated and analyzed in two directions: towards trauma and dissociation, and towards drive conflicts and repression. Thus can we retrace some of the footsteps of history in her therapy.

In his later foray into trauma Freud (1920) added a mechanistic set of concepts to his earlier ideas. He posited a stimulus barrier in the mind, which protected it from being overwhelmed by external stimuli, and he conceptualized trauma as involving the mind being presented with more external stimulation than it can handle, breaking through this stimulus barrier. The usual ways of processing and mastering stimuli are knocked out of commission. This is why upset is the opposite of trauma: to feel upset, you need a whole set of ego functions to produce and become aware of the feelings, while trauma begins at the point at which these ego functions shut down. It begins at a point beyond upset. The person will often describe feeling "numb," as well as having strange changes in their body awareness and perceptions. These are the outward, conscious signs of the shutting down of various functions, such as the integrative function, that usually construct, quite silently and quickly, our present experience. We see it very well in the incident when Cordelia is told of her mother's death. Suddenly something gives way, and everything is different. She experiences the punch in the stomach and invasion by fear and aggression and loss much more concretely and physically than would normally be the case with something that was merely upsetting. Here we see the partial loss of a number of ego functions—symbolizing and thinking processes—which now are unavailable, as reality assails Cordelia physically. Furst (1978) defined the stimulus barrier as involving inborn physiologic mechanisms, upon which later aspects such as defenses and other higher level functions are built. In a traumatic situation, the higher level functions are the first to fail, as the person is thrown back on more primitive defenses such as withdrawal, freezing, and numbing, and finally to the basic physiological mechanisms. If these fail, there is an unstoppable slide down into the acute, shattering traumatic response.

These ideas raise a number of questions. What do we need a stimulus barrier for? Clearly it's not just a matter of intensity, as a very loud noise or bright light might be unpleasant, but not traumatic. Complications like this have led many to reject the idea of the stimulus barrier as too mechanistic. Some have suggested that the key is the meaning of an event, such as helplessness, and the accompanying affects. But coming to terms with a situation of helplessness and experiencing and processing the accompanying feelings can actually be helpful, and certainly is not always traumatic. I gave an example of a man coming to terms with a terminal diagnosis, and feeling all the more alive for it, in my book on defenses (Fernando, 2009, pp. 91–93). So while meaning clearly plays a part, lack of preparation also seems important. Other authors, such as Van Der Kolk (2014), stress the importance of physical immobilization. There are of course traumas that do not strictly speaking involve this, although there is usually a freezing of action at least, as there was in Cordelia's case in that she could not eat or move. Actual physical immobilization does seem to increase the level of the trauma. Extreme fear, especially fear for one's life, is a key ingredient, and probably immobilization is related to this fear as well. However, one can be immobilized without being traumatized, if there is no fear, and one can fear for one's life without being traumatized, if there is time and space to deal with the idea. So here too, the factors of surprise and time and extreme fear are crucial. It is a combination of these factors that overwhelms the usual adaptive capacities of the person. As a preliminary working definition, we could say that the traumatic sequence involves being faced too quickly with too much that is frightful, leading to a sudden shutting down of the usual ways we process reality.

Triggers, Repetitions, and Conversion Symptoms

A number of things could trigger reactions related to her trauma in Cordelia. Once a customer unexpectedly got angry, attacking her verbally, and saying he did not want her business. She became quite panicked, much more than the actual situation demanded. She felt "like I was a little boat, cut loose from the mother ship." She made this comment without consciously meaning to refer to her actual mother, and only noticed the reference later. It may be thought that these sorts of triggering reactions, or at least their intensity and frequency, was a product of the therapy, and of our work on her trauma. I wondered myself if this was the case. But as we delved into both the trauma and Cordelia's life before therapy, it became clear that the largest part of her reactions were not a product of our work. In small ways and large in all of her relationships, she was triggered to re-experience aspects her trauma. One very large way was feeling compelled to leave relationships at the four year mark, without knowing why. Another example of the smaller triggers was when she heard of an accident in the city in which a car had been speeding and had gone out of control, seriously injuring three thirteen-year old children who had been walking on the sidewalk. She mentioned hearing about this and was quite shaken. "How will the parents find out?" was her first thought. "They wouldn't have any I.D. on them. The parents won't know till they don't come home." Again, it was only after we reflected on this, that she saw the similarity to what her father had said about her mother not coming home. She said her upset was because she was picturing what the parents would be feeling when they first realized that their child was dead. Again, surely a derivation from her own experience at age four.

Cordelia developed persistent stomach aches when going to school, beginning in the early elementary school years. Investigations could not find a cause. When she was a little older, one of the pains turned out to be appendicitis, and she was taken to hospital for an operation. "Before the operation I was sure I would die, and that no one could help me. None of them had any power to help me, so I asked the highest power, God, to help." The operation went well. In her early 20s Cordelia developed pains that traditional medicine was not able to help her with. One clinician had not only misdiagnosed her but said there was nothing that could be done to cure her. A couple of years later abdominal symptoms of different sorts returned. Since then she had tried all sorts of remedies both within and outside of mainstream medicine. She was losing weight when I saw her, and often would not feel like eating. She did not have the body image distortion or constant preoccupation with food and weight of someone with classical anorexia nervosa.

During her therapy, Cordelia developed discomfort in her abdomen, and was sure she had colon cancer and would die. A colonoscopy found nothing. She was pleased and surprised by this, and even more surprised by other feelings that came from the knowledge that she was not dying. She became sad and started crying. With this emotional release, the belly discomfort disappeared. It came back again later, and on other occasions there was this very interesting back and forth, with stomach symptoms disappearing as she became sad and cried, and then reappearing later. The anxious certainty that she was dying contained her upset about her mother's death, as well as expressing a powerful identification with her mother as she was dying. When Cordelia was told that she herself was not dying, this feeling seemed to have nowhere else to go, and came out directly as sadness. When she cried, and especially as she also linked it to her mother, her belly discomfort disappeared. A reaction like this does not mean that the symptom has no physical cause, as conversions of emotional reactions into physical ones often chose real pains to jump onto, a process that Breuer and Freud called somatic compliance. Often the physical cause will be a transitory one. When the emotion has jumped onto the symptom, the displaced emotions maintain it once the physical cause is no more. (In my clinical experience many—certainly not all, but many—symptoms that persist after infections and injuries are these sorts of conversion reactions.)

Let me go into a little bit more detail about another of Cordelia's conversion symptoms. She came in one session with a very painful right side. She had almost not been able to come to the appointment, she said. There were pains up her arm, a painful contracture of her hand, and vague pains going further down that side of her body. These later were hard to pin down, and the complex of areas and symptoms were hard to make sense of physically. It was hard to see how specific muscle, nerve, or spinal, or brain related problems were the cause. The whole story of how the symptoms had formed only emerged over a number of sessions. In this session Cordelia talked of the pain, which led to her crying, again a bit surprisingly to her, which led me to wonder about sadness leading to the pain. What she remembered was not this but that she had, the day before, been quite angry, fuming in fact, at her husband. Then the anger had disappeared, and the pain and muscle spasm of the hand had started. It had worsened through the night, and she had woken up in extreme pain. She only now made the connection between the disappearance of her anger and the physical symptom, which made her wonder if it was like wanting to hit him, to hit out with her hand especially. This horrified her. It wasn't the sort of thing she would do. In fact quite the opposite. But as she talked of this, the symptoms receded. It came back and then receded again as the session went on. As Cordelia felt her anger, or sadness, the symptoms would diminish, and then she would talk of other things, the feeling would disappear, and the pains and contracture would partially return. She was led to talk of her anger at me, as well as at her father, for not paying attention to her after her mother's death. Then of her lying in the hospital bed, beside but facing away from her mother, on the same side as her pains now were, when she visited her mother in the last weeks of her life. She remembered little from the months after the fateful night where her father had made his announcement of her death, but she did remember, she said, that she kept going to her father's bed at night and lying with him for comfort, on her side, cuddled up to him. When she left after that session what we had been talking of kept going through her mind, and over that day the symptoms cleared up completely.

Repression, Dissociation, and Ego Shut Down

It was phenomena such as those described in the analysis of Cordelia's right sided pains and contracture that informed Breuer and Freud's (1895) ideas about trauma leading to strangulated affect, expressed symbolically in bodily symptoms. They described how when the patient was led back to traumatic scenes where they had for various reasons not been able to express the emotional reaction that had started in them, and when they were able finally to give full emotional expression to their feelings, the physical symptoms would disappear. But Breuer and Freud had in the end very different explanations for what was going on. Breuer felt that the key was that the event happened while the patient was under the spell of a hypnoid state, in which their mind was divided in two, and thus their more regular mind could not take cognizance of their emotion, nor work it over. It remained split off until the work of analysis brought the emotions and thoughts and memories contained in the hypnoid state into the light of the person's more regular consciousness. Freud was respectful of his older collaborator and mentor's views in their joint publication, but even at this early stage stressed defense against unacceptable impulses and feelings, which led to them becoming, and remaining, unconscious. He stated that "It is not, indeed, that I have never had to do with symptoms which demonstrably arose during dissociated states of consciousness and were obliged for that reason to remain excluded from the ego. This was sometimes so in my cases as well; but I was able to show afterwards that the so-called hypnoid state owed its separation to the fact that in it a psychical group had come into effect which had previously been split off by defence. In short, I am unable to suppress a suspicion that somewhere or other the roots of hypnoid and defence hysteria come together, and that there the primary factor is defence. But I can say nothing about this" (p. 286).

If we look at how Cordelia described the appearance of her symptoms on her right side, we can perhaps walk in Freud's footsteps and see where he came up with his ideas. Cordelia felt angry, probably building to the strong wish to hit her husband, and then developed the pain in her arm and contracture of her hand, as she lost any consciousness of her anger. In more modern terminology, we would say that this was an instance of after repression or secondary repression. In his later work Freud detailed the primal repressions upon which these secondary repressions were based. In the material from Cordelia's therapy presented at the start of this chapter, the reader may recall that in the sessions described she was becoming aware of her own anger. She realized that maybe she had also been glad for her mother's death, and she realized that the intruders and murderers of whom she was afraid were also embodiments of her anger. In sessions before the ones described some very strong anger at her father, which had been powerfully repressed, had come to light. In fact the development of the arm and right sided symptoms were in part a product of this exploration. Cordelia had been in the beginnings of her Oedipal love for her father and wish to replace her mother, when her mother had died. She had been most sorely disappointed that her father had not put her in her mother's place after this sad event. In fact he had been in a surly and preoccupied state, even if he was still warm and loving in his own way, for instance by taking the children on walks where he showed them things in nature. Cordelia's anger, and of course the sexual wishes related to the Oedipal conflicts, had been repressed. As we were analyzing her anger at her father, we also saw that it was present towards myself, for not helping her enough and giving her enough guidance. However, Cordelia was not usually aware of this, and consciously felt quite an opposite set of feelings towards me. In all this, described in very brief terms here, there are many of the elements that Freud conceptualized in his later work, such as repression of powerful wishes, secondary repression of present day wishes that connect to these, the Oedipus complex, and displacement of these dynamics into the therapy and their transference onto the therapist, and even the fact that quick cures such as the disappearance of Cordelia's symptoms are partly based on the transference of these conflicts into the analysis (a transference cure).

In treating patients such as Cordelia, Freud saw emotional conflict everywhere, and he was not mistaken. There was a phase in Cordelia's therapy where anger at her father appeared in associations and dreams. There was a good deal of resistance to these feelings when they came up, and she would often find various reasons why perhaps we had been mistaken in this, or why she was wrong to be angry at her father. When this feeling was especially close to the surface and I interpreted it, she would get irritated at me. I have argued at length in my book on defenses

(2009, pp. 43–46 especially) that these sorts of reactions, of flashes of anger just as the defense is confronted, are evidence that what we are dealing with is what I have designated a **counterforce defense**. The therapy releases the aggression used in the repression, at least for a moment, when the repression is confronted. Most people are usually well aware of this sort of reaction outside of the clinical situation in the "sore spots" of the people close to them, which just have to be touched on lightly to elicit an angry response. This is one piece of evidence that repression is a form of internal defense that uses the power of the aggressive drive, in a somewhat modified form, to push powerful drives and feelings into the unconscious and keep them there. (Just to avoid confusion: I am describing the mechanism of repression. What is repressed—the object of repression—whether aggression, or something else, is a separate thing.) I bring this up here not in order to go at this point into the details of the dynamics of repression, which is one of these counterforce defenses, but to point to the sorts of reactions the analysis of which led Freud deep into the internal world of his patients. This repressed anger at her father was transferred by Cordelia onto me, but there too it was defended against, especially by a kind of internalization where she made things her fault, and held others blameless. In all of this, the illness and death of Cordelia's mother, and the trauma of hearing about it from her father, could be seen as important. But one can perhaps see how Freud could maintain that they gained their importance, their traumatic impact, and their power to influence her so many years after the events, by the drive conflicts and dynamics which had been triggered by them, and for which they served as a container.

In diving so deep into his patient's mental functioning, and into their unconscious, Freud made discoveries which were not only original but that are almost impossible to make. Both because of the strong emotional resistances against the realities unearthed, and because of their strangeness compared to what we usually think of as our mental functioning, these were not the sorts of discoveries that are made by many investigators independently of each other, when the time is ripe. In fact, from the moment Freud made them and up to the present day people, including many psychoanalysts, have been backing away from these findings. I want to make the point here, of how difficult these findings were to make, because it is often held against Freud, or seen as lamentable, that he did not appreciate the importance of trauma in the way that Janet and Breuer did. I think those who say he did not, and that he minimized dissociation in particular, are correct. But history works in convoluted ways. If Freud had better appreciated the importance and deeper nature of trauma and dissociation at the beginning of his psychological career, in the manner of a number of early investigators, he would no doubt have made further contributions to the topic. But if these had clouded his view of what he did discover, such as repression, childhood sexuality, and the primary process, and blocked his discovery and further investigations of them, we would certainly be much the poorer for it although, given how difficult these discoveries are to make, we might never have become aware of our poverty. As it was, Freud's discoveries in relation to the internal world did cloud his view to some extent when he revisited trauma later in his career. Our task now, I believe, is to investigate how Freud's monumental discoveries and the unique dynamics of trauma fit together, if we don't collapse one into the other.

In some of the modern literature on trauma (not all of it), these discoveries of Freud's are seen as either opposed to the new findings and ideas about trauma, or as having been superseded by them. For instance in a book on dissociation Elizabeth Howell (2005) says that these days we do not so much see repression in our patients as dissociation, and that the separation between id and ego is also a product of dissociation. In many recent works, the idea of repression is replaced by that of implicit memories. But repressions, of both the primal and secondary variety, are to be found everywhere in Cordelia's dynamics, as is dissociation. It may be objected that after all Cordelia was not so ill, or that her trauma was not so shattering, to display the preponderance of dissociation or implicit memories over repression seen in more severe cases. I would agree with the first part of this statement—Cordelia was not borderline, had stable and warm object relations, and her trauma was not so shattering as some can be. But I would argue that even in borderline disorders and shattering trauma repression plays its part, although the nature of repression is itself somewhat different in these situations. Examples will be presented later. One of the main themes of this book is that dissociation is just one—even though a central one—of the defenses used after trauma. Repression and other counterforce defenses play a prominent role, as do many other types of defenses such as obsessional ones.

The core of Cordelia's trauma was the announcement of her mother's death, and here we would expect dissociation to be present. What marks something out as trauma is that the nature of the event leads to a deeper regression (loss of normal function), and that annihilation anxieties (Hurvich, 2003) are triggered by either actual threats to life, or by experiences that are so shattering as to be felt as such. Thus there is a combination of a serious level of ego shutdown and of intense annihilation anxiety. Because of this, the event is not processed in the usual way, not integrated with other events, and not inserted into the usual flow of consciousness and memory. This is what Cordelia experienced as a little girl when she felt punched in the stomach, lost her breath, and felt a blackness enter into her. One basic ego function—the partial separation of bodily reactions from mental feelings and thoughts, with the subsequent emergence of symbolic thought—had clearly been put out of commission, leading to the concrete physical experiencing of her feelings. In fact it was as if they had been reduced to their physical and perceptual expression, with their more symbolic and psychical form having fled. And there was also the weakness of integration, coordination, abstraction, and differentiation of elements, all of which we pretty much take for granted as the background of regular experience, and only notice in their absence, when experience takes on strange qualities.

In post-traumatic defenses the person actively produces states similar to, and often based on, those passively suffered during the trauma, by shutting down various functions. A common and easily observed example of this is when during trauma a person will feel numb, as their processing of affects is shut down, and then they will actively (although usually not consciously) bring on the numbness in all sorts of later situations. Some of these may relate to the trauma, but others may not. I have had more than one seriously traumatized patient who could with little difficulty numb themselves and feel no pain when injured, or during dental procedures such as doing a root canal without anaesthetic. The connection of this active use of post-traumatic shutdown to the primary shutdown of the trauma became evident when, as we analyzed their traumas by undoing the repressions and dissociations that separated them off from the person's regular self, they had a much diminished ability to block off physical pain through numbing.

In Cordelia's case her sadness and crying seemed to come on unexpectedly, from somewhere else. Her physical reactions to being told her mother was not coming home, of loss of appetite, and a pain in her stomach, were still experienced as separate from the thoughts and feelings of the present time, unintegrated and floating off on their own. Her symptoms of not feeling like eating, and of pains in her stomach, acquired meanings, for instance in terms of identifying with her mother, or punishing herself, but at the core of these reactions sat the little bits and pieces of Cordelia's traumatic experience. These bits were not integrated with each other into a full experience with emotional reactions, physical feelings, perceptions, and thoughts all brought together. They rather lay shattered and scattered throughout Cordelia's life, and in her symptoms. These symptoms could be analyzed in either direction. As we saw with the symptom of the right sided pain, we could analyze the repressions and come to her present day anger, at her husband and towards me, which over time we could trace back to her anger at her father for not helping her, and not fulfilling her Oedipal wishes. But we could also analyze the symptoms to get to the split off, dissociated memories, of lying beside her mother as she was dying in hospital, and beside her father after he mother's death, and get to the sadness and confusion of those times. The blackness was the dissociated experience of death, the reality of which invaded her, even as it was also her repressed murderous wishes.

Fixation to Trauma

Cordelia's situation was in many ways balanced between external overwhelming and internal conflict. This is not uncommon, but is certainly not always the case. For instance if an intruder had come into the house when Cordelia was age four, and she had witnessed her mother being shot to death, the event itself would have been more shattering, and carried more weight, than whatever emotional conflicts would have become associated with it. On the other hand, we can easily imagine something with a greater weight on internal reactions, such as the birth of Cordelia's siblings. Here the external factor, of first seeing the baby in her mother's arms, and others admiring it, can be quite shocking for the child, but the angry, jealous reactions, and fears of being abandoned, dominate. However, the external event does not determine this by itself, but rather whether it causes a state of ego breakdown, which itself is determined by many internal and external factors. For Cordelia's trauma, I mentioned the lack of any preparation of Cordelia in terms of what was happening to her mother, as well as a traumatic hospitalization at age three and the quick succession of sibling births that put a strain on her and aroused her rage. On the other side of the ledger was the generally warm and loving relationship between Cordelia and her mother, the support and warmth of her very loving maternal grandparents, and her tendencies towards active mastery and relatedness to others, which she demonstrated almost from birth, and which were in evidence during her therapy.

Once ego breakdown takes place, we have a traumatic process. Is having the traumatic process enough to explain the later long-term effects, including such things as the repetitions of the trauma such as Cordelia's four year relationships, and her physical symptoms based on the event? What argues against this is that there is such a thing as **bland trauma**—in other words, trauma that heals naturally over time (Furst, 1978). This process takes a number of months. During this time there are the usual signs of trauma such as hyperarousal, dreams in which the event is relived, and phobic avoidances of certain things connected to the trauma. A patient of mine was, during the time she was in analysis with me, a passenger in a car that was hit by another car that was running a red light. The collision was completely unexpected (even more so as she was a passenger and was reading something when it happened), and pushed her car violently enough that my patient suffered a mild concussion. She had a reaction of looking back at the damage to her car, after she had stepped out of it, and not believing that the crumpled part of the car was real. This reaction of disbelief remained for a number of weeks, and was related to previous traumas, showing that it's hard to have a truly bland trauma. Still, there was spontaneous recovery. She had symptoms related to the incident, such as repetition in thought and dreams, and triggered reactions, that suggested that what had taken place was traumatic. These dreams and other repetitions have been conceptualized as attempts to belatedly process the event, which overwhelmed the ego in the first instance, and to put the pieces of it together into something resembling a normal memory. Over time, the incident had less impact on my patient, and the reactions disappeared. Bland traumas are relatively common – I have observed them on a number of occasions. We see these repetitions and dreams also in traumas that we treat, but in these cases they seem not to be able to achieve their goal. Why not? Why do people become fixated on traumas? It seems that there are mechanisms available to process overwhelming events that are beyond the abilities of the mind to immediately accommodate, whether they be surprise birthday parties or car accidents. Why in some instances do they not do their job?

Before engaging with this fundamental question, it may be worthwhile considering for a moment the fact that there are self healing processes that kick in after a disruptive event, even if it is of traumatic proportions. It is clear that these will be our friends in any therapy of trauma. In fact, we can briefly summarize trauma therapy as involving analyzing the things that have blocked this normal healing from going forward, and supporting the person as it unfolds in therapy. This spontaneous process of integrating the trauma can be compared to the spontaneous process of mourning, which also takes about 6–12 months, also involves disruption and painful feelings, and also restores better functioning and reengagement with the world. From the point of view of terminology, I am using the term and concept trauma to refer to the initial disruption, even if self-repair works and if the event is heard from no more. Some may say that such an event, for instance my patient's car accident, was not traumatic because it had no long-term consequences. Of course the word trauma can be used in many ways. The demarcation of what a concept refers to is arbitrary, in that it is a man made convention. But what is not arbitrary is that some demarcations allow us to see certain things better, and therefore to think more clearly, than others. Trauma is a specific example of this issue: delineating the concept trauma, differentiating it on the one hand from upset and other affects, and on the other from its long-term consequences, allows us, I would contend, to focus on this process and not confuse it with others. This can help us in a deeper exploration of the process, and also then help us to gain more accurate insight into its interactions, into the form of mental functioning that is left after trauma, and into such questions as what things lead to a fixation on the event.

So why does the self-healing fail, and fixation occur? Here are four possibilities: the trauma may be too overwhelming; the event may become entangled in powerful conflicts that are either already or subsequently repressed; the self-healing may be disrupted by events that

follow the initial trauma; and there may be constitutional or early acquired deficits that interfere with the healing process. Clinically, as we
try to analyze trauma we meet these factors in various guises.

The first resistances we meet when approaching a trauma are reluctance and avoidance (Kluft, 2000). These are so simple as to hardly
seem like true resistances, but an understanding of why they are used
leads deep into the true nature of trauma and post-traumatic mental
states. In fact, if we fail to meet reluctance and avoidance, we should be
led to wonder if what we are being presented with is something other
than trauma, or whether traumatic memory is being used for other
purposes. An example of this are the first sessions of many borderline
patients, in which they will talk at length and very insistently about the
traumas that they have suffered at the hands of their parents and others.
This is almost always a sign of weak repressions and flooding by drives
and internal emotions that are then projected onto external happenings.
Similarly, when repressions are weakened by analysis, or in other forms
of therapy, then internal drives and fantasies can emerge projected onto
the external world, as a trauma. This is the situation Freud faced with a
number of his patients, which led to him at first to propose that neurosis
was caused by sexual abuse, and then later abandoning this idea as he
realized that what he was dealing with were projected fantasies. While
Freud has been falsely accused of covering up sexual abuse in making
this reversal, in a more subtle way it led to a tendency for many decades
within psychoanalysis to not give trauma its due, by overgeneralizing
this common enough screening use of external events and trauma. These
dynamics are complex, and true trauma and the use of external reality as
a screen for internal conflicts are often intermixed. We can be helped in
finding our way by using as a guide the often shifting balance between
the most basic of post-traumatic defenses—avoidance, reluctance, and
doubt; and the presence of the most basic signs of the use of traumas as
screens—insistence and certainty.

In Cordelia's case, she did mention her trauma, and at times brought it
up herself, but usually would then go on to talk of other things. Her
avoidance was not so strong as can be found in some other traumas. The
traumatic memory served a screening function as well, in relation to
Oedipal wishes, in which the scene with her father and children and no
mother, expressed this wish. The avoidance would almost certainly have
been stronger in the hypothetical case I described, of her seeing her
mother shot and killed by an intruder. An example of a more extreme
trauma is found in a patient of mine, Peggy, who was sexually abused as
a young child, at seven and eight years of age, by her mother, who
suffered from paranoid schizophrenia. She was made to masturbate her
mother with her hand on a number of occasions, and her face was also
put onto her mother's genitals. Whenever I brought this up, in connection

with a dream, or a reaction of Peggy's, she would make a face, and at times she would cover her face. She almost never brought up the abuse herself, although I had of course learned of it from her, near the beginning of her therapy. There is much to be said about these reactions, and I will have more to say about Peggy's story later, but here I would just state that the strength of her avoidance I took to be a measure of the intensity of the overwhelming she suffered during her trauma. There was much less integration of the event into the narrative of her life compared to Cordelia, even though she was older when it occurred. It seemed that it was the strangeness and intensity of the event, and the extreme horror and disorientation associated with it, that especially led to this avoidance. At the time after each incident happened, this was one of the main things blocking the healing process. Right after it happened, as the incident was brought up in one way or another, the level of fear and confusion would lead to avoidance and blocking of any further processing of it. In the therapy there was a combination of strong avoidance—Peggy closing her eyes and saying "no!", and a very basic repression. She had at times in her life completely forgotten that the incidents had happened, and when I brought them up, she would get very angry at me in a specific manner, of a burst of quick anger, which I take to be a sign of the undoing of a repression. Thus something intrinsic to the trauma itself led to a blocking of the healing process, by avoidance and repression.

Along with the strength of the trauma was the fact that Peggy had to deal with ongoing difficulties and dangerous situations in relation to her mother. For instance her mother had once made a murderous attack against her father, and Peggy quite realistically feared for her own life at times. Most of the time her mother was in her own world, whispering to people only she saw or heard. Peggy would often be alone with her mother during the day when she was small, and later after school, before her more normal and stable father came home, and alone also at times on weekends or holidays, when her father was working at his business. In this kind of situation, processing of the traumatic incidents had to be put off till a later date, and the incidents themselves were largely compartmentalized, as Peggy dealt with the ongoing situation. So here we have two of the reasons that I listed as causing fixation to a trauma: the strength of the trauma itself, and the disruption of self-healing by other incidents and the general situation after the trauma. This second reason is always there in ongoing abuse and disruptive situations. Cordelia also had disruptions, of a lower level, following the trauma: her usually loving maternal grandparents were not as available emotionally, as they were devastated by the loss of their daughter, and her father also was more irritable and withdrawn. Even after the fact, they did not discuss the death, did not take the children to the funeral, and her father did not talk of her mother. It is hard enough to approach a very disruptive and upsetting reality and a four-year old, even one as spunky and bright as Cordelia, needs some help with this. But what Cordelia got was the opposite: a situation that taught avoidance of the upsetting reality.

To now look at the two other factors I mentioned—the trauma being caught up in various other conflicts, and the presence of constitutional or early acquired weaknesses: the connection to Oedipal conflicts, and conflicts over aggression were very much present in Cordelia's case, and have already been described. This type of entanglement is common and needs to be analyzed if the fixation on the trauma is to be reversed. I will be presenting details of a number of these sorts of entanglements, and the technical issues of how to work with them, in my clinical cases as we move through this book. In terms of constitutional factors, neither Cordelia nor Peggy had marked ego deficits, and in fact they were quite resilient young girls. This is also important to consider, in terms of how to approach the trauma. It was possible to bring up the traumas without engendering a sustained and uncontrollable regression with both these patients. In more unstable borderline cases, uncontrolled regression is very much to be expected, and it is best to first work on the ego weaknesses.

Overwhelming From Outside Versus Overwhelming From Inside

So far I have been presenting basic aspects of the traumatic process: external overwhelming leading to shutting down of important mental functions, dissociation based on this, the natural healing of this disordered area of the mind, and various things that can get in the way of this healing process, leading to a fixation on the trauma in the form of repetitions and symptoms. In order to venture further into the land of trauma, it will be necessary now to orient ourselves by using a basic distinction, between impingements from outside versus inside. Such a distinction may seem quaint or old fashioned, if not simply naive, in today's world of postmodern thought and socially constructed reality. The distinction between inside and outside, between reality and our own fantasies and models of reality, have become blurred over time to the point that now, at least in theoretical discourse, having any line at all can seem suspect. In such a confusing situation, lost in the wilds, not knowing whether reality even exists, it can be useful to fall back on an old fashioned orienting instrument as our compass: clinical experience. In situations of massive overwhelming by external forces, such as for instance the car accident of my patient I briefly mentioned, one observes characteristic features, such as continued repetition in dreams and flashbacks, dissociative defenses and reactions, phobic avoidances of similar situations, and triggering of reliving. These aftereffects are not there in situations of overwhelming from affects and drives. For instance, after an affect storm in which a borderline patient completely loses all rational and realistic responses, or in a severe temper tantrum by a toddler, in which their aggression completely overwhelms them, and there is a loss of language and many other capacities, one does not get these post-traumatic after effects. The child or patient may be quite shaken, the parents or therapist also, but the sorts of phobic avoidances and triggered reliving of the incident will not usually follow.

On the other hand, any traumatic incident would seem only to be traumatic based on the meaning given to it, showing that there is no external impingement independent of this internal meaning and understanding. We can think of what it meant to Cordelia that her mother was dead, which was different than if her father had told her, however abruptly, that her hamster was dead. Even the car accident of my other patient surely acquired its traumatic impact because of the fear of injury and especially of death. What I mean by internal impingement, however, is not thought and meaning, but rather the push of urgent internal forces—the drives and affects. In my book on defenses (2009) I asserted, and tried to demonstrate through clinical examples, that the defenses directed against the drives, and at times strong affects as well, involved a powerful counterforce against the drive or affect. I argued, following Heinz Hartmann (1948, 1950, 1953), that this counterforce was formed from partially neutralized aggression, used to push these forces out of conscious awareness and to erect a stable barrier to keep them there. The best known counterforce defense is repression, but reaction formation and isolation also use a counterforce, in these cases bound together with other processes in a **compound defense**.

One of the main themes of my defense book was that different defenses from those used against inner urges were usually used against aspects of external reality that were distressing. I referred to these as **attentional defenses,** because instead of a powerful intrapsychic counterforce they used combinations of suppression and normal attentional processes to look away from a distressing reality. The best known of these attentional defenses is denial. This differentiation was well enough known before the conceptual discussions in my book, but the differing mechanisms had not been explored carefully, and linked to the nature of what was defended against. This is crucial: one can turn attention away from reality or a memory of reality but in the case of a drive, which pushes powerfully from the interior of the mind, this will not do, and a counterforce is necessary.

In the early days of analysis, when drive/defense conflicts were thought of as the primary determinants of neurosis, denial was deemed a more primitive defense. Anna Freud's book "The ego and the mechanisms of defense" (1936) devoted much of its space to describing attentional defenses such as denial in thought, word, and action, restriction of the ego, and identification with the aggressor. But she in the end describes these as pre-stages of defense, again suggesting that they do the work for a while, when the child is immature, until more mature defenses such as repression and reaction formation come into play. The idea that denial and associated defenses are more primitive or immature also comes from the observation that they are used as a replacement for weak or failing repressions in borderline and psychotic disorders. To take an extreme example, Edith Jacobson (1957), in an early paper on denial and repression, described the case of a psychotic man who expressed his wish to have sex with his mother. This would seem to be a direct expression of what are usually deeply repressed Oedipal wishes, due to the breakdown of primal repression because of the psychosis. But Jacobson noted that in fact this patient was defending against wishes to be passively sexually loved by his father. These wishes were felt as extremely dangerous because they were linked to a wish to be castrated, and the active heterosexual wishes were focused on as a defense. Here attention was shifted to one fragment of a deeper id drive in order to defend against another. As the counterforce defense of repression crumbled in this psychotic man, he was forced to fall back on an attentional defense to try to hold dangerous wishes at bay. Obviously in a case such as this the denial was immature and ineffective, and repression or something similar would have done a better job. Jacobson used this example to point out the different mechanisms of the two defenses but she also, in this paper and in more detail later (1964), described the normal use of denial, to deal with everyday reality. In the regular course of things counterforce defenses such as repression do the heavy lifting in dealing with drive conflicts and the associated memories and affects. Denial defenses merely serve secondary purposes in these cases, but are used as the primary defenses against distressing external realities. The fact is that we all use denial and other attentional defenses to keep distressing realities out of awareness. The denial of the narcissism and lack of love of a parent is a common example of what I have called primal denial.

In attempting to frame a general theory of defenses, I (2009, also see 2013 for a shorter summary) divided them into the two broad categories of counterforce defenses and attentional defenses, and also suggested that each defense could be present as a powerful, stable primal defense, and also as a more transitory secondary defense. As an example, my patient Peggy developed primal denials of the self involvement and bizarreness of her psychotic mother. These protected her from the overwhelming fear and sadness that a full awareness of what her mother was like would have engendered. Later, more transitory secondary denials were based on this basic primal one. Unfortunately, a defense such as Peggy's primal denial may not be flexible and under the person's control, so that she then would deny very distressing characteristics of other people, which led her to get into, and stay in, a disastrous marriage to a psychopath—a history I will describe in later chapters.

All of us have, along with our basic primal repressions, a store of what I (2009, pp. 91–93) have referred to as **universal primal denials**. These involve the denial of our fragility, of our helplessness in the face of chance and necessity, of the limitations in the amount of love and attention anyone can give us, or we them, and of our own death. These denials are not abstract, but have a concrete individual aspect in each of us. Their existence does not preclude intellectual acknowledgement of these unpleasant realities, and even emotional awareness. But denial is kept up at some level, shored up by religious beliefs, sentimental feelings, unconscious fantasies, and other methods. It would be dangerous to have a complete denial of our vulnerability or death, and in fact universal primal denials involve a balancing (not conscious) of practical acceptance of these realities, so that our actions will be reasonably realistic, and yet the maintenance of a feeling of invulnerability all the same, which allows us to act and live without being overwhelmed by dread. Universal primal denials protect our mental stability. This becomes clear when they are challenged by events—such as when Cordelia's father told her that her mother would not be coming home, or Peggy's mother took her to bed and forced her to perform various sexual acts. Or when my patient was suddenly jolted and pushed around as her car was hit by another car, jumped through the air, and came to an abrupt stop. Each of these very different events share the fact that they shattered some part of the person's basic primal denial. Observation suggests that universal primal denials are complex, flexible, and dynamic structures, largely unconscious, which usually bend and change rather than breaking in the face of events. Given a bit of time and some support, they can adapt. As I had described previously, if Cordelia's parents had told her about her mother's illness, she would have become upset, and her primal denials would have been shaken, but they would have had a chance to adapt. It is only the abrupt shattering of a primal denial that leads to the ego shutdown that we call trauma. Primal denials are one part of the stimulus barrier that is shattered in trauma.

While primal denial is a specific way in which my theory of defenses connects with trauma, the more general connection is simply that the theory is based on a view, with much clinical support, that the mind faces in two very different directions: inwards towards the drives and powerful affects, and outwards, towards incoming external stimuli. Our conscious mind is closely tied to external perception, as Freud (1923) pointed out. Even our own thoughts are at first unconscious, and can only become conscious once they have been linked to external perceptions, whether sounds or visual symbols. These two different directions that the mind faces involve different inputs, different levels of conscious perception of the input, different ways of dealing with the input, including different methods of processing and different defenses, and different forms of primal defenses that build up protective but permeable barriers to too much impingement. I also argued in my defense book that the two ways the mind faces both contribute to its functioning, and that the defenses primarily used in each direction—counterforce defenses against the inside, attentional defenses against the outside—and the dynamics built upon them, are both of importance. They each enter as independent factors into various mental dynamics, symptoms, and behaviours. And I would say the same of the most extreme of external impingements—trauma, which leads to **primary dissociation** of sets of memories, feelings and thoughts, that survive in split off islands of the mind. *Trauma and post-traumatic mental functioning enter as independent factors into mental dynamics. They cannot be reduced to other factors, such as drive conflicts or developmental deprivations, nor can these other factors be reduced to trauma.*

Having established a framework, related to forms of impingement and types of defenses, related to trauma, and having looked at trauma in terms of its causes and consequences, including normal healing processes and how these get derailed, it is time now to dive into our main topic—the nature of post-traumatic mental functioning, which I have designated as the zero process.

Chapter 2

Trauma, The Zero Process, and The Construction of Reality

Joyce was a number of years into an analysis with me, during which we had dealt with sexual abuse from her childhood and relationship difficulties in her adult life. She had always remembered a time when she was travelling as a young adult and had visited the house of an older and very successful colleague, in order to follow up on a position that he may have been able to offer her. She had said previously that he had made a sexual advance on her, cornering her in his back yard. She had run away, and never contacted him again—in fact had gone directly back home, which was quite a long trip from where she was. She had passed over this time rather quickly when it had come up, being vague about what had happened, and generally avoided talking about it. But at this point in the therapy, we had been led back to that time by certain reactions of Joyce's in the present day, as well as discrepancies in her story, especially related to the timing of events and of when she came back. She herself seemed driven to make sense of what had happened, but then as she approached it would find herself backing off and avoiding the topic.

In this session, I point out to Joyce that as she brought up this incident she started saying, "I don't know," at the end of almost every sentence. This proclamation had been much in evidence as we approached the most overwhelming part of Joyce's earlier childhood traumas of sexual abuse, and the statement increased in frequency as we came closer to those core memories. I have observed this particular statement, and other ones such as "maybe," in similar circumstances in many patients, and see it as a form of denial with regard to these traumatic memories: an energetic turning away from what is seen.

I say that her saying "I don't know" might be an indication that something further had happened. Over a number of sessions, we establish that this man had put his hand on her knee and then had invited her to walk in his garden.

"So what happened then?" I ask.

"I just remember running away."

"So he must have tried something further."

DOI: 10.4324/9781003283218-3

"Maybe. I don't know. I just don't know."

"Well, see what you think of. Remember how in looking at the abuse by [her abuser in childhood] it seemed you didn't remember anything, but as you paid attention to it, more and more came up?"

A look of what seemed like a mixture of anger and anxiety passed over Joyce's face. "Nooo, Nooo" she said, combining the word no and a moan in one utterance.

"You look upset"

"I feel you're pushing me. You're pulling me into this, into looking at this, but it's not good."

Previously, when we were looking at her childhood abuse, Joyce had said she felt I was "bothering" her with questions and interpretations. We had traced this back to her feeling of being "bothered" by her abuser. As we talked at this later point about the incident with the colleague, she complained a number of times about me and others "pulling" her into things.

Over the next few weeks Joyce developed bronchitis-like symptoms and a feeling that she was having trouble breathing. In one session I said, "I wonder if he grabbed you and pulled you?"

"No. I don't know!"

"But if we look at your reactions, it might be that he grabbed you in the garden as you tried to run away. You said he was a very big man. Maybe he was on top of you and you could not breathe."

"I am feeling the weight of him on me. But I don't see him."

"What do you see?"

"Nooo, Nooo." Joyce moaned. You're pulling me and pushing me now. It's not good."

"So it feels like it's now?"

"It is now. You're just pushing me too hard and I can't breathe. There's a burning in my throat. It hurts a lot."

"Did he perhaps grab your throat? Or perhaps force oral sex on you?"

"No. I know that wasn't it."

"So he probably grabbed you and pulled you. Then what?"

"The grass was soft on my back. I just said that. I don't know really. How do I know?"

"Well, you just said it was soft on your back. Maybe in the end you were on your back. What did you see?"

"I didn't see him. I didn't see anyone."

"But if you felt the soft grass, you must have been on your back, so he must have caught you."

"Noooo, Nooo. I don't know. You're pushing me too. I feel I can't breathe. I see the sky and the flowers, that's all. It's all very quiet." Joyce said all this in a quite angry tone.

The analysis of this incident took a number of months and involved the analysis also of the repression of the time after, when Joyce was in a daze.

When this first appeared, we thought it was a single incident of rape, from which she had run away.

What emerged over a number of years of therapy was something even worse, and also somewhat different from what we first thought. This part of Joyce's story will be told at the end of chapter three, in the section on dissociative identity disorder (DID). I have introduced these fragments from our work together at this point because they demonstrate a number of characteristics of post-traumatic memories, and post-traumatic mental functioning more generally. I presented these excerpts from Joyce's analysis in a paper on the zero process (2012a, 2012b), in order to illustrate them concretely. What was surprising to me was that each time I presented the paper my official discussant, or some members of the audience in the discussion, focused on other aspects. One discussant, in New York at the annual meeting of the American Psychoanalytic Association, questioned whether Joyce's memories represented a true event, or a compromise formation, a kind of screen for repressed conflicts and transference fantasies. Of course, this is a possibility. In fact, further analysis showed the distortions and repressing and screening functions of the memories from the rape, in relation especially to what came afterwards. But I did wonder why this was main theme of his discussion. A number of other commentators, at other presentations, have concentrated on the enactment between myself and Joyce, where I do end up pushing her, and she ends up being overwhelmed. These commentators saw my behaviour as the cause for Joyce's feelings of being trapped. I would not hold out these sessions as models of good technique in the analysis of trauma but again, I was struck by this being the focus of comments. A book length treatment of the topic allows each of these important issues to be taken up in turn, while still leaving space for what this example was meant to do, which is to illustrate something about the nature of the zero process. And clarifying the nature of the zero process sheds light on such issues as screen trauma and clinical technique. So, I would ask the reader to put these other questions in brackets for now while we look into the nature of post-traumatic mental functioning.

Traumatic Memories and The Construction of Reality

The characteristics of the sort of reliving displayed by Joyce are well known and well described by those who work with trauma and by those who have suffered from it. The memory behaves more like a perception or immediate experience. It has the sensory intensity of experience, but also the lack of any distance between the observer and the memory. The pieces of experience as they occur are also not well integrated into a linear narrative. For Joyce the feel of the grass on her back, the weight of the man on top of her making it hard to breathe, the sight of the sky and flowers, and the extreme fear, were all felt in their full immediacy, but all somewhat separate from each other. In fact, they were more intense than what a regular perception or experience may be. There are many reasons for this. One that was important in this case, and quite common generally, was that the memory served to screen even more deeply repressed traumatic memories. Leaving screening on one side, other factors leading to the intensity of the reliving included of course the intensity of the original experience itself, and the shutting down of a number of ego functions, especially abstraction and integration, during the trauma. This has been well understood by many trauma theorists: that the lack of processing of the original experience is what leads to its intensity and staying power. But it is worth noting that processing is a general term, which covers many different mental actions. These different actions also have a hierarchical and sequential aspect. By which I mean that certain actions have to be performed before other functions can be brought to bear on the experience. An example relevant to trauma is that adding symbolic language, a narrative, and relation to the self to memories of an event are later stage actions. A good deal of processing, a good number of different mental actions, must be performed before you have a set of memories that have even the possibility of being connected to language and a narrative. These actions are usually performed so quickly in regular experience that we do not notice them, and we assume that the end product of these actions is direct, unmediated experience, which can then be connected to words and become an autobiographical memory. I would propose to refer to the summation of these basic mental actions as the first order construction of the present moment or of present experience. Trauma exposes the existence of this first-order construction by interfering with it and, in extreme cases, shutting it down completely.

Normally we sample a small amount of the incoming perceptual stimuli, comparing it to our expectations and models of the world, to construct our experience. This all takes place below the threshold of awareness. Integration of different sensory modalities and pieces of experience across time is an example of this subthreshold activity. We see the lack of it in Joyce's bits and pieces of experience as they emerged from repression in the sessions described. Not so often commented upon, but also important, is the work of differentiation. As an example, in regular experience feelings are differentiated one from the other, one differentiates oneself and one's experience from that of others, and different sensory modalities, even as they are integrated, are also differentiated. When describing his feeling at the height of a physical abuse situation from early childhood, one of my patients described it as "sadfear". He did not mean feeling sad and afraid at the same time, he said, but rather a different and strange feeling, where they were part of one unitary feeling—his fear of his out of control parent, and sadness that they were behaving in this way—thus demonstrating the breakdown of the usual process of differentiation during his trauma. In fact so different was the feeling that at first he could not find any word for it, and it took some work for him to be able to perceive the components as separate enough for him to find a name. Identification with the aggressor, so common following trauma, is used to defend against helplessness, but is also based on the lack of self/other differentiation at the height of trauma. (Ferenczi (1933) described this aspect long ago.) Our immediate present experience is a product of the subtle and ongoing, but completely unrecognized and taken for granted, interplay between integration and differentiation. When these processes are deficient, experience takes on strange qualities, of fragmentation but also of lack of the usual boundaries between self, other, and various features of perception and feeling.

Of the functions that fail during the traumatic process one of the most consequential is a superordinate one, which Hartmann (1950) called the organizing function. While its name may give the impression of something highly intellectual, it proceeds much more quickly than conscious thought or the intellectual functions. Its work is to give each function its place and importance in a fast, dynamic, and flexible manner. A well running organizing function would be able to put thought aside in many areas so that automatized and rote functions, which are much more efficient, can manage things, calling up consciousness and thought only when useful. This organization and ordering of various functions breaks down during trauma. A number of other mental actions are also impaired or completely shut down, among them abstraction and the linking of the perception to previous ones and to the person's models of the world more generally. But if this was all that occurred in trauma, then we would have memories that were fragmented, unorganized, overly concrete, and not well put together in other ways. They would still behave like regular memories—they could be retrieved, and would tell a rather strange and imperfect tale of what had happened, reflecting the person's mental state during the trauma. What actually transpires is different—and decisive. While what is left after trauma behave like memories in the sense that they are retained over time, in most other ways they behave much more like present experiences. Joyce did not remember her rape in the usual way, she lived it as a present experience. Once the experience was set going, she could not control it. She could not for instance stop it, and look back at some earlier part of it she had just thought of, as we could with a regular memory, even a memory of a terrifying incident. I first gave the name zero process to this type of post-traumatic functioning in my book on defenses (2009). (The term was suggested to me by Dr. William Shantz at a meeting of the Toronto chapter of the International Neuropsychoanalysis Association, when I presented my ideas there (Matthis & Deutsch, 2005).) I decided on the term zero process because this connected it with the primary and secondary processes, as one of the three great regions of the mind, or ways in which the mind functions. I felt the name also suggested more of an addition, rather than a replacement, of what had been discovered about the primary process in development, in neurosis, and in so much of regular functioning, by Freud and other analysts.

It has been evident since the beginning of scientific work on trauma that traumatic memories behave very much like experiences. However, in thinking of the zero process, it has only dawned on me slowly just how important it is to think of post-traumatic functioning not just as memories that are very intense and thus mimic experiences, but rather to understand that the core of post-traumatic functioning really is, at the psychical level, not a set of memories at all. They have the characteristic of memory of being retained over time, but in other ways they behave like an experience. Or, more accurately, something like Joyce's reactions are not regular experiences, they are a kind of raw, only partially processed, experience. More than this, they are experience before it has happened, stopped short in the middle of its construction by the traumatic process. By using our understanding of the traumatic process, as something that leads to the shutting down of ego actions involved in the first-order construction of experience, we can make sense of the seemingly senseless idea of a memory/experience that has not yet happened. Because the bits and pieces of these zero process memories, for instance Joyce's memories of her rape, have not been used to construct the experience, we can quite rightly say that, at the psychical level, the experience has not yet happened, in the usual meaning of an experience that has happened to us and can then be remembered. What Joyce had were zero process proto-memories: such stuff as not only dreams and fantasies, but experience itself, are made on. Her experience of the trauma had not yet been fully made. It existed as a potential, and in that sense it was still in the future, although when triggered portions of the traumatic memory would play out as an immediate present experience. Conceptualizing the nature of the zero process as a present/future experience, about to happen, at times happening, but never happening fully enough to be encoded into more regular long-term memory, can seem at first enigmatic. But it is an enigma that, if unravelled and properly understood conceptually leads, as I hope to demonstrate, to the unravelling of many of the other enigmas surrounding trauma.

Joyce's dramatic reliving is only one way in which the zero process expresses itself. It lives as another reality, a reality that is always about to happen, or happening. As a more common example, we can take Cordelia's reaction when someone was sick, of pushing all sorts of remedies on them, and getting angry at them for not being more active in attending to their health and following her advice. This type of pushiness was not a general character trait of hers. Rather, it was informed by the other reality, a zero process reality, that had existed for her since her mother's illness and death. In this reality the person was about to die, and regular medicine and regular treatments were not going to work, just as they hadn't worked for Cordelia's mother. Quick action and desperate measures had to be taken, as it was a life and death situation. Also, Cordelia was angry at this dying person for not taking care of themselves and for leaving her all alone. A number of Cordelia's other reactions, for instance her stomach pains, loss of appetite, and loss of weight, also related to this other reality. This is how the zero process usually presents: as sets of physical and mental reactions which are thought by the person and those around them to relate to the present reality, but which are actually an expression of the unprocessed traumatic one in which part of them unknowingly dwells.

A dramatic example of this second reality was presented by William Niederland (1981) in his description of a former inmate of a Nazi death camp: "one of my survivor patients told me that at the time of liberation from the concentration camp his weight was down to 94 lbs. and he looked like a 'plucked chicken.' Though he is now of normal weight and appearance, he cannot be sure—he told me—that he has not the looks of a plucked chicken still today, and with great regularity he refuses to leave his home, in order not to be seen by other people" (p. 417). Another of Niederland's (1965) patients had been diagnosed as schizophrenic because he seemed to have the delusion of freezing, even in hot weather, and would dress in layers of clothing, and shiver in the office. Other aspects of his interactions in the therapy did not seem schizophrenic to Niederland and as he stuck with him in therapy the patient began to thaw out and not feel so cold. A dream depicted him near or at the North Pole, his bed a block of ice or a refrigerator, surrounded by the ice, cold, and darkness of a seemingly endless night. When dawn finally came, some people walked in and out of the room where he lay. Niederland was led to ask his patient, in analyzing this dream, if he had ever actually had an episode of freezing. The patient asked his parents, who were surprised, and said they had left the widow in his bedroom open on a very cold day, and he had almost frozen to death, and had to be thawed out. He was taken to hospital, where he acquired a pneumonia and took quite a while to recover. This had happened when he was less than a year old. Upon the patient hearing of this episode, the therapeutic outcome was immediate and sustained, without any of the seeming psychosis returning.

The quick cure demonstrated by Niederland's freezing patient seems almost magical. It certainly differs from the more common stubbornness of post-traumatic symptoms, even as we uncover their roots. This is one of the enigmas around trauma—the quick cures and the interminable therapies. The quick cures seem to relate to single incidents or sets of incidents, often from a very young age, which are not part of ongoing traumatic overwhelming and chronic stress. Another example of such a cure from the early analytic literature is provided by a young patient whose analysis was described by Alvin Frank (1969). He was a boy of five whose transference behaviour and obsessive interest in being tied up led his analyst to question the boy's mother. She confessed with shame that for one month when he was eight months old she had been severely depressed. During this time she had strapped him into his high chair and left him like this for the entire day. Upon being informed of this by his analyst the boy immediately demanded to talk to his mother. He confronted her and got her to tell him what had happened. Though he recovered no distinct memory of that time, this interchange was followed by rapid changes. He showed an increased ability to distinguish wishful fantasy from reality and he was able to work through the theme of being tied up, which was interwoven with fantasies from each psychosexual stage, but which had stubbornly persisted through earlier attempts to analyze it. This demonstrates an important clinical finding: that one needs to analyze and make real the zero process fragments that have been caught up in or expressed in other conflicts and fantasies, before these other conflicts can be usefully analyzed. It also brings up the issue of very early trauma and memories—in this case and Niederland's, no perceptual memories were recovered. And yet both these patients were clearly being influenced by a second reality, without knowing it. One way to further get our bearings in relation to this strange second reality is to compare it to the one that was first investigated by Freud: the primary process.

The Zero Process, the Primary Process, and the Secondary Process

By all clinical indications, the core of the zero process functions as an experience. Freud (1925), in conceptualizing the perceptual apparatus, compared it to a slate that is wiped clean each time, ready for new impressions. Memory, by contrast, involves the creation of a more permanent formation. As the input from a sensory receptor moves into the mind, it is analyzed first for basic qualities, and then for more holistic, gestalt aspects. These later are more obviously related to past experience, for instance a specific face or a voice, but they are only the continuation of a process of analysis of the input and construction of the experience which begins with very basic qualities. By the time we have what we think of as our immediate experience of reality, a good deal of this processing has already taken place. Our conscious experience takes place as we combine the outcome of this processing with memories and models. Slights of hand and illusions rely on the fact that our expectations create our experience. And of course from this point on, processing of the experience still continues.

What we know is that trauma disrupts this processing of incoming sensory data at various points. An upsetting or unpleasant experience may be resisted in the sense of trying not to recognize it and making it real—the sort of experience where the person will say, "this can't be happening!" At a higher level of disruption you get the breakdown of the basic processing of the event, as described previously, leading to changes in level of consciousness, to lack of integration, etc. Some combination of the suddenness of the event and of the breakdown of universal primal denials leading to annihilation anxiety, causes a shutdown of the processing of incoming stimuli, along with the shutdown of other ego functions. Why external overwhelming leads to this kind of shutdown is not a question I think we have a good answer for, at least in terms of ultimate causation, even though we know some neurological correlates. The answer may have to be sought more at the evolutionary than at the functional psychological level. It is clear that the basic traumatic response, including the formation of memories that behave more like experiences, is present at least among mammals, and perhaps in somewhat different form in some other animals with complex nervous systems. There are various theories related to freezing responses, over activation, and the adaptiveness of creating indelible memories of dangerous situations. Powerful learning after only a single event is useful in extreme circumstances, and it may be that in trauma this mechanism, which we see in stressful and frightening events, overshoots the mark, leading to a kind of single event learning that is not so adaptive.

The key aspect of the zero process to understand is that the realities related to trauma are present at all times, as a second reality that the person has to respond to. Because we become more directly aware of zero process memories when reliving is triggered, as happened in the example with Joyce, it may be tempting to see them as more regular but very powerful memories that are evoked by experiences. Many observations argue against this view. When one analyzes more deeply, one finds that the person is in fact always reacting in subtle ways to this reality. Or, to phrase it more accurately, some of their actions, feelings, and beliefs are from that part of them that still lives in the other, traumatic, reality. Along with her present reality, Cordelia lived in a world where a woman was losing weight, had pains in her belly, had no appetite, and had a deadly disease that the doctors could not cure. This reality expressed itself in Cordelia's physical symptoms, feelings, and behaviour towards others. Peggy, my patient with the paranoid schizophrenic mother mentioned in the last chapter, was full of humour, connected to others emotionally, and had a lively interest in the world. At the same time she also lived in fear, was jumpy, and easily spooked and panicked. As we uncovered the depths of this, she admitted that she always lived in fear, feeling separate from the people around her, embarrassed and ashamed and feeling that she was living in a world no one knew about or suspected, given her lively personality. This she did not consciously link to the time living with her mother, in fear for her life and embarrassed and confused by her mother's crazy behaviour, as she walked around in see-through nightgowns whispering to unseen people, but it was clearly an outgrowth of this other reality. One thing worth emphasizing is that the present day reality was not just a cover or false. Peggy really was connected in a deep way with people, had a genuine sense of humour, and took genuine pleasure in art and her intellectual interests. It did not strike me at all as a false self in the present covering over her true reality. Rather, Peggy lived in two realities, as did Cordelia, and Joyce for that matter, as I will describe below when we go a bit further into her story. This distinguishes zero process functioning from schizoid and psychotic disorders where there really is a thin layer of normal functioning covering over a deeper break with reality, based on global, rather than focal, deficits in important ego functions. Niederland's freezing patient was misdiagnosed as psychotic because of the bizarreness of his symptom, but Niederland saw the more regular functioning and contact with reality, which proved not to be a facade but a part of him, alongside which the patient also lived in the cold and frozen reality of his early trauma.

The reality of zero process experiencing is brought home by the physiological changes (for instance changes in blood pressure, in need for vision correction, etc.) that have been measured in patients with dissociative identity disorder (DID, formerly called multiple personality disorder), between the different personalities or alters (Putnam, 1989; Loewenstein & Ross, 1992). It is this disorder especially that brings out the fact of another reality. Kluft (2013), one of the foremost authorities on DID, has referred to it as not a multiple personality disorder but rather a multiple reality disorder. There in fact seems to be a continuous activation of the perceptual end of the mental apparatus, giving the sense of the experience continuing. From early investigators on, the fact that the trauma takes up part of the perceptual apparatus, and that the person is thus not able to fully live in and react to the present, has been described—for instance by Janet (quoted in Van der Kolk, 2014, pp. 181–183) and in Breuer's descriptions of his patient Anna O (Breuer & Freud, 1895).

Brain facts for some reason feel more real to many people than psychological facts, so here is one that relates to this aspect of the zero process: at an annual meeting of the International Neuropsychoanalysis Society on "minding the body" in 2011, Heather Berlin presented a case of a DID patient one of whose personalities (alters) was blind. Functional imaging studies on the patient when the blind alter was in control showed significant changes in, among other places, the primary visual cortex (V1). This surprised the investigators, and I and others in the audience found it striking as well. We would have expected changes in areas involved in assessing perceptions, or in integrating them, but not in the cortical area that visual input first comes into, and which processes the basic characteristics of the image. Audience members asked about further investigations of the patient, but were told that she was in therapy and as the alters integrated the blindness, as well as the brain imaging changes in V1, disappeared. This is a powerful demonstration of the two way feedback and feedforward routes in the brain and the mind. One short-hand way of conceptualizing zero process memories is that they involve the invasion of the perceptual apparatus of the mind by characteristics of memory: what should be a largely blank slate for incoming stimuli from outside and inside the body to present themselves on, acquires some more long-term structures that properly should be part of the memory systems.

While many of the affects, thoughts, and body reactions related to reliving of the trauma are reactions to perception which stays as a perpetual present or just about to happen moment, truncated or unfinished actions are also present, and also important. They are part of the unprocessed past that lives in the present. This is especially shown by the importance of performing specific physical actions in the therapy of, and recovery from, trauma. The intention to act, when it becomes part of the zero process, has not only its characteristics of remaining a perpetual present, but also of remaining unintegrated with other actions and perceptions and judgements. The work of therapy is to bring this integration about. While often perceptions and feelings seem to dominate the patient's trauma awareness, this may be partly because of the close tie of our conscious awareness with these. We should not forget that the intention to act, and actions themselves, are one of the key components of our mental functioning, and thus of the zero process traumatic moments that become frozen in a perpetual present.

Post-traumatic mental functioning has at times been conflated with the deeper emotional aspects of the mind that Freud called the primary process. More recently, full knowledge of the primary process has been obscured as it has been absorbed into object relations theory and a broadened idea of infancy, development, and trauma. Freud first introduced the idea of the primary process and described its characteristics in the Interpretation of Dreams (1900), where he demonstrated how, through the method of free association, he could not only reveal hidden wishes and forgotten memories, but also a form of mental functioning that was different from that of which we are usually aware. By comparing the manifest dream with the repressed latent dream thoughts, memories, and fantasies uncovered through the method of free association, Freud showed that the original thoughts had been subject to a number of changes. These transformations, which occurred in all cases, and also in the formation of symptoms, jokes, and artistic productions, led Freud to infer that the thoughts had been subjected in the unconscious to novel mental processes. He called this the primary process, implying that it was there from the start, only to be later overlaid by the more reality-oriented and organized secondary process.

Freud's idea of the primary process was an experience distant one, involving inference from observations. Dreams are not pure primary process, any more than psychotic processes are. What we actually see is a complex combination of diverse influences. Similarly Joyce's reactions and our interactions in the sessions I described earlier were not a pure expression of the zero process. Rather, as her defenses gave way and as the traumatic memories emerged, we could catch a glimpse of some characteristics of the zero process more clearly than is usually the case. Certain experience distant concepts, if well fashioned and a good representation of important processes that we cannot directly observe, can have enormous explanatory power. I believe both the primary process, the zero process, and the idea of different forms of mental functioning more generally, are such concepts. As a further demonstration of this explanatory power, I will try to demonstrate in chapter four how looking at borderline disorders in terms of the primary process can be quite clarifying.

To now compare: in the primary process there is an unceasing movement. Freud (1900) conceptualized that psychic energy in the primary process is freely mobile, always trying for a path of discharge, as compared to the secondary process, where the energy is bound. In the primary process energy and interest are easily displaced from one thing to another, and different contents can condense to form one image. Time does not effect the strength of wishes, or the nature of the contents of the primary process more generally, which led Freud to call the primary process timeless. There is no distinction made between fantasies and reality. We can observe a number of these processes at work in Cordelia's aggressive fantasies and death wishes towards her parents, which had been repressed at an early age. These wishes were generally projected onto other figures, such as the dog that landed on the ground and lunged at her in a dream, or the men who she was always afraid were breaking into her home. Here we see displacement, as well as condensation of sexual and aggressive wishes in the invading men. Fantasies of murder scare her and make Cordelia feel as guilty as if she had actually done the deed, showing the lack of distinction between fantasy and reality. The wishes and fantasies were certainly unaffected by time, as fresh when they emerged in therapy as they were when she was a young child. The core of Cordelia's zero process was also untouched by time—for instance she was always losing weight, always having stomach trouble. But the core of the zero process is timeless in a more frozen or mechanically repetitive manner. There is none of the ceaseless movement, also none of the displacement and condensation, seen in the primary process. Rather there is a moment or a series of moments, frozen in time, endlessly running in a loop. As one of my other traumatized patients expressed it: "I just start to get upset and run through the reactions and feelings, once it starts. And then it's like it rewinds like a videotape, ready to start up again. It's like I have no control over it once it starts, and no control knowing it's going to begin again sometime." The wishes and contents of the primary process are outside of time, and uninfluenced by it, or by the further experiences and learning that come with time. The frozen experiences of the zero process are uninfluenced by time, but they contain a piece of time in a sequenced state, ready to unfold. This sequencing is absent from the primary process.

The primary process treats all psychic events as real, and in this respect there is a defective sense of reality. Since the zero process involves a past reality living out as if it were a present reality, it does involve reality testing and a connection with reality, just one that is not judged correctly as part of the past. The primary process especially confuses fantasies and reality, while the zero process confuses past traumatic realities with present realities. It treats memories as present realities, while the primary process treats fantasies as present realities.

While energies in the id, where the primary process reigns, are freely mobile and strive for discharge as they quickly jump from one thing to another, and those in the secondary process are more bound and measured in their movement, the zero process is a different thing altogether. On the one hand, there is certainly not easy movement and displacement—rather a fixed pattern of perception and affect and action and bodily changes is activated and lived out. We might say that the energies are rigidly bound, having only one form of discharge—a fixed repetition. On the other hand, unlike the rational control in relation to means and goals imposed by the secondary process, the zero process has the restless striving for immediate discharge associated with the primary process. But the channels of discharge are tightly constrained. The id is powered by the drives of sexuality and aggression, which strive for discharge. The zero process is powered by not yet fully formed experience, which strives to finish forming and to become real.

To what are we to attribute the drive-like character of the core contents of the zero process, that lead to the repetition of aspects of the trauma? Freud (1920) posited the death instinct. Some analytic authors from the generations after Freud (Lipin, 1963; Greenacre, 1967; Cohen, 1980) talked instead of a maturational drive, and a need to complete the formation of the traumatic experience. This is closer to my ideas, although I would say the drive is not developmental but functional. It seems to be a compulsion built into the functioning of the mind related to the construction of the present moment. We certainly know this tendency well enough, as we see it in our need to finish processing even relatively non-traumatic situations such as a surprise birthday party that is a truly unexpected, in which case we will find our mind going back over the moments of surprise, and those leading up to it, and also feeling again the surprise. It shows itself very powerful and persistent after trauma. Only in a metaphorical sense can this be conceptualized as a drive to return to an earlier state of things, as Freud suggested in formulating the death drive. It is really an attempt to finish a normal piece of the mind's functional work, and this unfinished business happens to relate to a past situation. Nor is it developmental, in the way that this word is normally used. It is rather an aspect of the present functioning of the mind and brain, and in that sense functional rather than developmental. Of course every function can be effected by developmental changes, and it would be more than a little interesting to inquire into how this functional **zero process drive** may change through phases of development.

Despite the disagreements, I am in agreement with Freud, Lipin, Greenacre, and Cohen in one important respect: I think that the pull to repeat traumas is based on more than just ego actions such as trying to undo the helplessness of the trauma, and turn passive suffering into action. This something more is the push from a certain type of drive-like force, with some similarities to the sexual and aggressive drives of the id, but some differences as well. I think this idea, really a finding, derived from work with trauma and analysis of the repetition tendency, is a true addition to our understanding of what the mind contains and of how the mind works. I will discuss this further in chapter three, on the zero process drives and zero process defenses, but will now continue with the comparison of the different types of mental functioning.

What about thinking? Generally thinking, the linking together of various memories to build up a model of the world, to make plans, connections, etc. is seen as an organized, secondary process function belonging to the ego. In the id there is a much more primitive form of primary process thinking, with connections between elements being made because of superficial similarities, elements being condensed together also without regard for deeper similarities, and a very concrete symbolism related to the body especially, taking the place of the language based symbols of the secondary process. In saying that this form of thinking is more primitive, I mean merely that it does not involve binding of energies and does not take account of reality. In fact, even minor creative thinking requires the use of primary process forms of thought, not just in artistic creativity but in scientific work as well. What of the zero process? Its concrete, experiential, and repetitive nature would seem to argue against there being any zero process thinking at all, but there are in fact two forms of thinking related to the zero process. The first is not zero process thinking per se but rather thinking occasioned by it. It is well known among those who work with trauma that the particular theories that are formed immediately following the trauma about why it happened, what it means etc., have enormous influence over a person's life ever after. Often these theories can be seen to have a defensive function, such as taking on responsibility for bringing the trauma about as a defense against feelings of helplessness. However, their persistence and large influence can also be traced to the fact that they are related to the other reality, the traumatic zero process one, that is always active in the person's life, so they too are always active. They make sure that the person is adapting to the past, but psychically still present, traumatic reality, even as the person also tries to adapt to the actual present. Thus these theories owe their strength to the fact that they are about something real, not just a possibility or a fantasy. We know that the reality is objectively in the past, but psychically it is still present, and the theories get their power from this fact. These theories share the immediacy, persistence, and repetitiveness of the zero process, because they are linked to it. They belong on a continuum with another form of thinking related to the zero process: since the zero process freezes certain actions taken at the time of trauma, into a constantly repeating present reality, then thoughts occurring just as the trauma is gathering steam, or at its height, which might be fragments of judgement as the ego shuts down, or just as the person comes out of the trauma, will be part of the repetitive core of the zero process. These will be as much a part of traumatic repetition as zero process feelings, body reactions, actions, and perceptions. As an example Peggy had a disgust reaction and judgements about herself as bad and ugly, related to her reaction to being forced to touch and then smelling her mother's genitals, when she was seven and eight years old. These were true zero process thoughts, which had all the reality and immediacy of the zero process, and existed quite untouched by time or experience, alongside very different self judgements.

One further point of comparison: the area of the id where the primary process reigns would seem to be much larger than areas of zero process functioning. The id has not just all the repressed drive conflicts, but also a huge amount of fantasies and wishes and memories, etc. By comparison the zero process core consists of just a few frozen traumatic incidents. But the area of the id is an internal area of potentially active wishes, memories, affects, etc. The area the zero process occupies is not really an internal area but an external one—another reality. And, even though zero process realities often are not as evident as in flashbacks or in Joyce's reliving, they are constantly influencing our reactions to reality, our bodily feelings, and our actions, or the actions we do not take. Thus this small area has an outsized influence on many things. Let us proceed now to list a few of these things, to get a sense of the range of this influence.

Some Applications: Mourning, Intergenerational Transmission of Trauma, and Internal Objects

Many things can have a zero process version. As an example we could take mourning. Volkan (2014) describes perennial mourning in a number of his patients. For these patients the mourning is never over and the lost person is ever present. The mourner does not develop depression, but continues endlessly to engage with the object. Volkan describes a patient who talked to his dead brother in his car driving to and from work, even though in other ways his reality testing was fine. He describes such patients dreaming endlessly about the person, but the dream always ends before the conflict is resolved. What is going on in perennial mourning? It would seem to be a different way of getting stuck in mourning, as compared to depression. The comparison between depression and perennial mourning is instructive of the nature of the zero process, as compared to the primary process. In depression the mourning is repressed, because there are irresolvable conflicts, often over angry feelings towards, and negative thoughts and memories about, the person who has been lost. The mourning requires revisiting these wishes, thoughts, and memories, but since they are under powerful repression, the mourning itself is dragged into the unconscious. At this point, in order to preserve the lost person, the whole process is internalized, the patient identifies with the lost object, and directs their hatred now at themselves, in the role of the object. As Freud says, "the shadow of the object fell upon the ego" (1917, p. 249). Because of the repression, the person no longer has access to certain memories and feelings about the lost person and so the mourning, which needs this access, is brought to a halt, and the whole process comes to share in the timelessness and interminable nature of the primary process. In the cases of perennial mourning that I have seen, the loss was caught up in a traumatic process, and frozen in time. There is the endless repetition of perceptual and feelings elements related to the lost person. The mourner does not develop melancholia, but continues endlessly to engage with the object. In perennial mourning, which could also be called zero process mourning, the accent falls on an ever present and ever repeated experience, which is what marks it out as a zero process phenomenon. It has a different kind of timelessness than depression—more repetitive of specific experiences, with the accent especially falling on the perceptual and affective aspects, while in depression drive and mood aspects, especially the continued aggressive attacks on the self, predominate.

In my experience of patients with perennial mourning, the traumatic overwhelming seemed to come as they were already mourning. They were in the painful phase of mourning where they had recognized the loss, when it became too much and they became traumatically overwhelmed.

Theirs was a more internal trauma, although related to an external loss. (This is an opportunity to clarify what it means to say that a trauma involves external overwhelming. Clearly it can be a judgement about reality that proves overwhelming and too much for the person, and thus tied to internal feelings. But this is different from, and behaves differently from, overwhelming from drives or the powerful affects associated with them.) With the trauma and the zero process memories tied to the pain of loss, the defensive maneuver is to stay at that point, and avoid the next phase, the release phase of mourning, where the painful recognition that the loss is real leads to a partial de-investment from the lost object. In regular mourning there is a constant back and forth between these two phases, of painful recognition of loss, and then of de-investment. At first the person stuck in perennial mourning may seem as if they are doing the work of mourning, and confronting the pain, but over time it becomes clear that this is a traumatic fixation used for defensive purposes, to avoid the final emotional letting go of the lost object. Pain is OK, release is not. (Cordelia's was a mixed case as her first trauma, the one I have described, was before the mourning, but she also became traumatically overwhelmed later as the aloneness and loss sunk in, and thus did display some of the characteristics of perennial mourning—something I will describe in the next chapter.)

There has been much interest in, and much written about, the intergenerational transmission of trauma. From a zero process point of view the key point is that what is passed down are not memories or feelings or sets of beliefs, but a reality. The traumatized parent who draws the child into their world of past trauma has been described by many authors, especially in relation to the Holocaust, but also other traumas, individual and collective (Bergmann & Jucovy, 1982; Brenner, 2014; Volkan, 2015). A number of concepts proposed in relation to intergenerational transmission convey the sense of a piece of reality being passed down and carried by the child. Volkan (2015) introduced the concept of a representation that is deposited in the child by the parent, while Kestenberg (1980) talked of transposition, in which the reality of the trauma that the adult suffered and the reality of the child's life are transposed. I think it is significant that these authors felt the need to come up with separate conceptualizations to point to something quite different from more regular mental actions. The concept of depositing suggests something concrete that is given over to the child, while Kestenberg (1980) specifically differentiated transposition from more regular primary/secondary process mechanisms such as identification. The intergenerational transmission of trauma involves zero process characteristics and dynamics.

Treatment for such people needs to involve confrontation with reality. Grubrich-Simitis (2010) talks of the need for her patients, children of holocaust survivors, to confront and test the reality of what happened to their parents. She notes that action in reality, and testing of reality, had very specific therapeutic effects. "The perception, recognition, and historicization of the Holocaust as external reality, together with the step-by-step process of symbolization in the context of the Auschwitz visits, proved to be essential preconditions for the progressive development of signal anxiety" (p. 61). These technical recommendations stem from the nature of the zero process as well, and show that its power passes down through the generations, an important finding also in considering sociohistorical issues.

Another psychological phenomenon that bridges the individual and the socio-historical realms are internal parents and internal others more generally, and especially the most complex and consequential of these—the superego. Our understanding of internal objects could be clarified quite a bit by applying the idea of **zero process objects**. We would expect these to be linked to specific traumatic incidents, to have strong perceptual and action aspects, and to have a repetitive sort of interaction with others, or a set of reactions. Introjects generally have this character. The idea of the introject, as an internalization of an external object relation, that resides within the person and yet confronts them as something external, has not been well explained in terms of its mechanism of formation and functioning. It can be contrasted with identification, in which our self and actions take on characteristics of those we love, or hate; and also with object representations, which are built up from regular memories and their abstraction and integration, belonging to the primary and secondary processes.

There is a continuum between more regular internal objects and zero process objects, depending on the contribution of each type of functioning. However, because of the drive like quality of zero process structures, which strive to become a full present experience, introjects seem to have, and in fact do have, a motivation independent of both the id drives and of the regular ego interests of a person. As an example, Peggy's traumatic interactions with her psychotic mother had been partly internalized as a scary mother introject. In her case this did not mean that she was aware most of the time of this attacking and crazy inner mother, but she was aware of its effects. She felt in danger and felt she was always trying to get away from something. She was also, and in contrast, adventurous and full of fun, which is how those around her largely experienced her, as she lived in these two worlds. The key zero process aspects of this inner mother were that she stood apart from Peggy, had an independent existence and behaviour that Peggy could not control, and that her behaviour consisted of specific repetitive actions that were linked to the traumas that Peggy had suffered at her mother's hands.

Zero process objects play a central role in the building up of the inner world of human objects. Not that the inner object world is simply a zero process world—far from it. There are the aforementioned identifications and self and object representations based on more regular, rather than zero process, memories, and the part played by drive (sexual and aggressive) investment in these. There is also the important part played by narcissism in its investment in the self and objects, whether regular or zero process, in forming our ideals and ideologies. However, what give inner objects and the inner object world a sense of reality as a present experience, and a sense of agency as something that acts independently of the person, are the zero process memories and zero process drives that reside within them. In this book, I will be working out the nature of the zero process and of zero process drives and defenses, and using these ideas to explore zero process objects in pathological and symptomatic phenomena, such as the alters of dissociative identity disorder, discussed in chapter three, internal objects in borderline disorders discussed in chapter four, and therapeutic techniques for working with zero process objects, described in chapter five.

The view of internal objects informed by the zero process extends beyond these topics, however. It has many applications. The internal object world and the superego are not just pathological phenomena. They are at the core of what it means to be human: central to normal development, to social interactions and group formation, and are also indispensable to an understanding of the evolution of the human mind. But in order to mine the possibilities of the application of zero process theory to these topics it will be necessary first to develop the theory to some depth. This enterprise—the development of zero process theory through the investigation of symptoms and dynamics as they appear in the clinical situation—is the work of this book. A book to follow will build on these findings to investigate the place of the zero process in normal individual development, in social structures, and in evolutionary processes.

And now—on with our exploration of the zero process! To round out our discussion of the basic nature of the zero process, let's move to a consideration of that complex, sometimes controversial, yet always fascinating, topic: memory.

A Trip Down Memory Lane

My patient Peggy was an adult in her 30s when the memories of the sexual abuse by her mother arose in her. The memories did not flood back all at once, but rather she would have flashes of something seen, or felt, or smelt. She did not get far in remembering all that had happened because she found these shards of memory too distressing, and generally avoided thinking further about them. The immediate trigger for the first memories that returned was some drawing that Peggy was doing in a class. Once she realized that she had been abused, she would be led to think about it despite herself, and more details came back. She also realized that she had never really forgotten about these incidents, but had avoided thinking about them to the point that they largely disappeared from view. This memory recovery happened a number of years before Peggy came to see me for therapy.

Peggy did not explicitly come to me to work on the abuse, but rather because of anxiety and feeling she could not put her life together after a psychologically abusive relationship. She mentioned the sexual abuse only later, as she was talking about her life with her mother, and about how she always tried to escape from the house during the day, when her father was not there. She found the abuse was very hard to talk about and each time she talked of it, she would mention a few details, put her hands over her face, and change the topic, or at least slide to other details of life with her mother. She had remembered many details of other parts of her mother's reactions, all quite disturbing, throughout her life, but tried not to think of these either. It was not at all clear to her whether she had ever completely repressed the memory of the sexual abuse, or had partially repressed it and then, through avoidance, had managed not to think about the time when it had occurred.

Peggy remembers that her mother had taken her to bed and had masturbated Peggy and gotten Peggy to masturbate her. She remembers, with a lot of disgust, the smell of her mother's vagina and the feel of the warm, large body against hers. She remembers looking at the crib of her younger sister in her room, as if she were fixating on that when something else was happening. These memories come as little shards: the smell, an image, and the fear and disgust and other feelings. The placement of the memory in time was at first not given, perhaps for defensive reasons, but also because this sort of age placement does not belong to concrete memory fragments such as these. I had assumed, by the way she described herself, and their obscurity, that these were very early memories. I was surprised to find Peggy knew very well when they had happened, and that it was later than I had thought. Her mother had come to her bed to do this when she was between seven and eight. Here we can see at least two types of memories: the concrete traumatic memory fragments, and the knowledge memory (what is called semantic memory) of when the things took place. When the semantic memory was accessed, Peggy would then also access various regular perceptual memories (what are variously called episodic, explicit, or autobiographical memories), a third type of memory. There are other forms of memory as well. One of the interesting discoveries of psychology and neuroscience over the last few decades has been the existence of these many different forms of memory, differentiable at the psychological and at the neuroanatomical level. Let's look a little further into Peggy's story and her memories, which can serve as examples of the various forms of memory and their dynamic interrelations.

Much of Peggy's psychotherapy, which was conducted at a twice a week frequency, sitting up, concerned her present situation, her relationship with her three children, her continuing problems with her ex-husband, and the history of that very troubled marriage. Peggy was thriving in her early adulthood. She had an active social life, did well in university, travelled, and developed her artistic and intellectual interests. She met her husband, Ted, in her mid 20s, and was not as much impressed with him as with some of the other men she met and dated. He was not very good socially, although he could be quite charming at times, and at others was very good at making her feel sorry for him and want to take care of him. The wish, in fact pressured need, to take care of people who were suffering was very strong in Peggy.

It seems that her ex-husband, Ted, was very good at doing just what he needed to do to keep Peggy interested, from those first meetings and on into their marriage, even as she never really developed true deep feelings for him. There was a reason for the lack of deep feelings, and it wasn't because of Peggy's inability to have these feelings. It was something about Ted. He was charming, narcissistic, and manipulative of those around him. He had no real warmth and seemed in the end only interested in power and money. Peggy was vulnerable because of her background, but she was not uniquely vulnerable. Ted got all sorts of businesspeople and professionals to join him in ventures, often getting them to give up other excellent positions or opportunities. He induced them to do this with promises of money or positions, promises that he never kept. He got rich through these ventures, but no one else seemed to profit. He slept with the wives of associates even as he was partnering with them on ventures and was still married to Peggy. Much of this Peggy only learned later, in talking to some of these people. Ted also made sure he got rich at Peggy's expense. He ingratiated himself with her father, who came to admire him so much that he made him the executor of his will. He had a good deal of money, and after his death Ted, using his position as executor, started moving money into his businesses. The bank alerted Peggy, but Ted was too canny, too good a liar, and too aggressive in pursuing his goals to let this stop him. Through manipulations, lies, getting some of Peggy's relatives on his side, the use of aggressive lawyers, and using the court proceedings to drain Peggy of all of her resources, both emotional and financial, Ted acquired almost all of Peggy's share of her considerable inheritance during and through the divorce proceedings.

I saw Peggy many years after the divorce. Ted's attacks on Peggy had not stopped with the breakup. Even after having gotten most of the money, he harassed her in the courts and through his manipulation of their children. Our therapy really started to make headway in dealing with Peggy's depression when we realized that she especially became depressed over a period of four months each year, which were the four months leading up to the time when Ted had left her. After the date of his leaving passed each year, she would feel much better—less depressed, and more connected to the world and the people in it. Ted had worked hard to make his leaving as painful as possible, by keeping Peggy guessing and saying terrible things to her, but then getting her to play the devoted wife at dinner parties she hosted for business associates, where he played the perfect, doting husband. Beyond his own self interest and getting what he wanted out of the marriage, his seemed to enjoy making Peggy suffer. "I was like a zombie during that time at the end. I just wanted to shout out at the dinners, 'he's leaving me, it's all a lie,' but I never did. I just smiled and made the perfect dinner and played along." The connections of all this with what had happened with her mother were legion, but the marriage was a trauma in its own right as well. In fact it was many traumas, both single incidents, such as times when Ted verbally, physically, or sexually attacked her, and the induction of an atmosphere of chronic tension and fear. This ongoing layering of one trauma, and one form of trauma, on top of another was also a way in which what went on in the marriage resembled what had gone one with Peggy and her mother in her childhood. I will now present some details from a few sessions to give the flavour of how the various traumas and memories emerged in Peggy's therapy.

This sequence of sessions starts near the end of one of Peggy's yearly four month depressive periods, at a point where we had figured out the connection with Ted's leaving her. In a session, she begins by expressing her frustration, and surprise, that Ted would not give any money for the kids. These are his grandchildren, and hers, who are having some troubles and need to go to a camp that their mother (Peggy's daughter) cannot afford. "It just makes me so angry that he won't pay. It's hard to understand why he won't do it. He's got so much money. They really could use it. He knows it and he had said before that he would pay."

"I'm surprised you're so surprised. Wouldn't it be more surprising if he came through?"

"I know. I know. But I guess I still want something different from him, even though I know it will never come. I still hope he will be different. Will care."

Peggy then wonders about a link to her mother. I say that maybe it's not that they are that similar, but that she used the same ways of dealing with the situations. She may, I suggest, have had similar hopes for a normal mother. This leads Peggy to remark on how she has so few memories of her mother from childhood. Her memories are all of playing outside.

"But because we have been talking about it something, a memory, came back to me. It just came to me a few days ago. I remember a dream of tugging at her leg to get her attention. Pulling at her. She seems so big. I must have been very young. It gives me a terrible feeling, so lonely." At this point, Peggy shudders and seems quite overtaken by the image and feelings. I have an uncanny feeling myself, of something strange.

"She didn't notice me; she was looking up to the air, whispering. I couldn't get her attention. It was actually kind of creepy. In the dream I was looking up at her, pulling and pulling trying to get her attention in the hallway. I don't remember something like that exactly, but when I think of the dream it seems like something like that must have happened a lot. It feels very familiar." When she says this, Peggy gives a demonstration of what she remembers, looking up and whispering with her mouth largely closed, as her mother did as she talked to unseen hallucinations. "I guess she just couldn't give me much normal attention."

"Did she sometimes pay attention to you in a normal way?"

"not so much, not so often"

"But that suggests that she did sometimes. Can you remember one time where you had a regular sort of interaction?"

"She could be very sweet and smile ... But no, I can't. But it must have happened sometimes." Peggy looks sad.

"Why? It's possible it did, but we can't take that for granted."

"I remember her wanting to hug me. I would always be pulling away. It was like I was a doll or something that she wanted to hug. She often wanted me. To hold me. But it wasn't like I was a person, just a rag doll." Here too, there is a creepy feeling in the air, which I think we both feel and I see on Peggy's face. As these memories are flooding in she says, rather surprisingly, "I don't remember anything." I point out to her maybe she means she doesn't want to remember anything. She is silent.

She talks a bit more of her mother's behaviour, but then she recounts a memory that she has always remembered and has recounted previously in the therapy.

"I was very young. Maybe three or four. I had run from the house, and I remember the trucks coming at me down the road. That was before we moved to the farm. I still have that fear if I'm driving and a truck comes up beside me. I can't pass trucks on the highway."

I say that it must have been pretty bad with her mother for her to leave like that. Or maybe her mother just wasn't watching her.

Peggy then recollects her embarrassment when her mother came to the high school—how intense that was. She cringes. I'm struck by the abrupt shift to this time in adolescence. It is a feature of Peggy's therapy, these shifts. She thinks again of pulling at her mother, who was whispering to the people in the air. I wonder if she had to push her mother away so forcefully because she was afraid that she would become crazy like her. She says that when she knew what her mother had, she was much more understanding and less angry. But that wasn't till university. Before that she just thought she was "retarded and crazy." She tried to kill her dad. She thinks she tried to strangle him and smother him while he slept, and he got a lock for his door. She explains that her mother then slept in the big room. What I wonder about at this point is how could he not be worried about the girls, if she was crazy and had tried to kill him. I ask about this and she says, oh, no, she left them alone. But I bring up that she did sexually abuse her. Was this in the daytime, which is what I had thought? And she says she came to her bed at night. "Maybe it was when my father would not do it with her." It strikes me that there is more to the sexual abuse, and that she might have changed the time of it to protect her beloved father. But if it was at night, and he slept behind a lock, she might have resented that he did not keep her safe. As she talks of the sexual abuse, she cringes.

At the next session, Peggy starts by saying, "I can't remember what my mother called me. That seems strange, since I have a good memory. Did my mother called me anything?" She then again thinks of her whispering, of her being "out of it," of how she as a little girl burnt her hands on a curling iron that had been left on, and wonders if that is why her father sent her mother to the psychiatric hospital. As we talk of the details of this, it is clear that in fact she was sent away probably a year later. I wonder if Peggy is finding ways to protect her beloved father from her own accusations that he did not protect her adequately from her mother. She remembers seeing her sister come home after her birth, looking through the banisters, at age three. She remembers what her mom wore. She wasn't sure if it was a real memory. But when she much later told the details to her father, including her mother's dress, he had confirmed them. Her mother was sent to the psychiatric hospital for shock therapy. Then her father took her out after a few months even though the psychiatrists advised against it. He couldn't fully face the truth about her. Peggy was four when she came back, and they lived in a house in the city from age four to eight. Her mother was very vacant. Even reading her letters to her father before they were married, they were vacant. Her answers were very limited, while his were fulsome and descriptive, and he asked her to give him more details of her life, coaching her. Peggy as a child was mainly embarrassed by her, as she walked around in her see-through night gowns.

At the next session, Peggy's mood is noticeably better. She says this, and I say I can see it, and point out the timing, as this was when Ted would have left. Peggy talks of how he behaved towards her, how he really tried to break her. "I always had a positive relationship to myself, but he almost crushed that. It took me a few years to recover but I did. He worked on destroying that belief in myself. He would be so very sweet to me in public, and everyone would think we were the perfect couple. Then he would turn cold as soon as we stepped through the door into our house." He was really after the money—that was what he got from others, and he worked on Peggy's father, who really loved him. He charmed him, and then her sister as well, to get the properties. He systematically isolated Peggy, even charming the therapist that she was seeing, and that they both saw as a couple, who thought he was just so perfect, and wanted Peggy to be the perfect housewife to him. Peggy talks of how she herself was always very related to people, that she was mischievous and would get into trouble, but was always very well liked by her teachers; always had good friends.

At the session following, the better mood continues. Peggy says it's my amazing job at therapy, but I point out each year it happens at this time. This leads, through talking about her abandonment by her husband, to her mother who also left her abandoned, and I wonder about the meaning of this reliving, over the four months; whether there is perhaps some connection to her mother. She talks of her memory of being alone, walking down the street with the trucks coming at her. She still gets scared of trucks. She must have been taken in by a nice lady. "I still remember her. She had beautiful vases in her house, lots of them. I collect exactly that type." (In a later session Peggy showed me a photo on her phone of all the vases lined up on a shelf at her place, beautifully arranged.) "I remember sitting there, so happy. The sunlight shining through the window and the vases." She remembers a nice warm feeling being with the woman. She felt safe with her. She does not remember how she got home. No one ever told her the story of this outing. "I never told anyone about that, or the rest of the memory, so it's not like one of those memories that you've been told about. But I've always remembered it."

I ask her if someone came to get her, but she says she remembers nothing of that. Only the peaceful feeling of being in this woman's house. Maybe she had given Peggy something to eat, she says.

Then a shift: when she was an infant, Peggy says, for her first year she was taken care of by "aunt Sally," really a distant cousin of her father's, Peggy thinks. She was very nice, motherly. "She really saved me." Later, after her marriage had fallen apart, Peggy had visited her and asked her about her mother. Sally said her mother had not prepared anything for the birth. Peggy's father gave Sally a blank cheque and she bought the crib and other things that were needed. When she went to pick Peggy up in the morning, she described how her mother would just be sitting there, with picture books all around her on the floor, and when she dropped her off at the end of the day, she would still be there, seemingly not having moved all day. The house was all dirty. This leads me to ask about her being then left with her mother. Peggy says aunt Sally just took her for the day. I try to ask her if Sally mentioned what happened then, when she was dropped off, and her father wasn't there. Who would have cleaned up her diaper, who would have fed her, if it was just her and her mother? Peggy gets a bit confused, talks quickly and talks over me, saying that her father must have come home soon after, even though at other times she had said her father worked long hours at the business. She tries to brush over this. She says that after her first year, her father moved the family to a different city, to start a new business. So after the first year she had many babysitters, her father had told her, but none stayed very long. They could not deal with her mother, who would get paranoid and aggressive with them. She thinks of how the place was filthy, and of how she would have been toilet trained—by her father or the babysitters, most likely. Her mother was just "out of it."

There were incidents. There was the one where Peggy picked up the hot hair curling iron, when she was very young, and burned her hand very badly. She remembers her father shouting at her mother for this. "Maybe this is why he sent her away," she says again. I point out that he had sent her away later, when Peggy was about four. But then she ended up coming back. He brought her back against the doctor's advice. The psychiatrist had said she wasn't ready yet. They later moved to the country. She talks of cleaning her place (in the present) to make it OK. to invite people over. But it's never clean enough. What does that mean? I have had the sense that it's not the terrible mess she sometimes says it is. In other sessions she has agreed, and shown me photos of a nice clean place, with clutter. But then the sense that it's too much of a mess comes over her. It strikes me that she is describing the other reality that she lives in—the reality of the times when she was alone in the dirty home with her embarrassing, scary, crazy mother.

Peggy comes in the next session and says that after the last session, she was haunted by memories of her mother's eyes. "She had a look that's hard to describe." Peggy puts her hands over her face as she talks about it, and she looks spooked when she opens her eyes. Spooked and scared. I ask if perhaps the eyes were narrowed, or angry? She says it was when she was angry and complaining. They were like daggers, but also crazy. Strange and murderous. Peggy imitates her mother's voice, which is raspy and menacing—something mean and something crazy about it. "I haven't seen those eyes in anyone else, ever." Not in her husband, not in other people who were angry. We are then led to talk about her husband when she talks of her depression and of how it's funny that she gets depressed at the time of year when he left, because he was awful for three years before, having affairs, starting around the time her father died. She talks of feeling so guilty that she was not there when her father died, even though she could not have known. She still held herself responsible. "I'm haunted by it," she says. Especially by her last phone call to him, as he sounded so weak, and died hours later.

In these excerpts from Peggy's therapy her search for knowledge of her past can be seen struggling with a wish to avoid memories of her past.

This was not a battle that took place only when she entered therapy. After her marriage breakup she went to see aunt Sally, who had taken care of her as an infant, with the intention of finding out what it had been like for her, and what her mother had been like. Before this, in university, once she learned about schizophrenia, she read more about it in order to come to understand what had really been wrong with her mother. After her husband left her, she talked on a number of occasions to other people whom he had dealt with, and whom he had cheated, to share their experiences. She was searching for both facts and explanations. She kept going back, even as she hated them, to the memories of the sexual abuse by her mother. But she had also partially repressed these memories. Even as she tried to remember, she tried to forget. She always tried to run outside, to get away from her mother, beginning perhaps with her trek on the road with trucks when she was very young, to playing outside on the farm when she was older, to her interest in all things beautiful, and her strong intellectual curiosity, by which she tried to escape the scary, ugly, depressing world of her mother and of her husband. In the sessions she continued this running away as she would go only so far in a topic and then flit to another one, sometimes just as I started to make a comment. At a deeper level, in these sessions we can see the evidence of Peggy's repression of her blaming her father for not protecting her from her mother. Some of her distortions of her memories, and times where she changed the topic, related to this repression.

In all these dynamics various forms of memory played their part. In his early work on the ego, Hartmann (1939, 1950) talked of memory as one of the primary autonomous ego functions, along with thinking, motility, perception, and a number of others. What Hartmann meant by primary autonomy was that these functions had a constitutional basis and developmental timetable. This does not mean that they are not effected by experience and conflict, only that they are not created by them. As an example of this influence, perceptual abilities would seem to be especially hard wired and yet if a child is born with cataracts that are not removed and thus lacks visual input, their visual cortex, and thus at the psychological level their visual function, will hardly develop at all, and in fact if the cataracts are removed too late, the function may never develop normally. Thus environmental input even here is crucial. But, in an average expectable environment (Hartmann, 1939) such functions as memory and perception will develop largely independently of experience, although of course they will very quickly get drawn into conflicts. The very formation of a fantasy or a wish or a conflict depends on the development of such primary autonomous functions as perception, motility, memory, and thinking.

Ideas about memory have played an important part in the exploration of trauma. All of those who have proposed theories about the nature of trauma have stressed special forms of memory, from the early work of Janet, Breuer, and Freud, to the present. There are two main groups of ideas, not mutually exclusive, relating memory and trauma. The first declares that during trauma some forms of memory, usually normal episodic or explicit memory, are put out of commission, so that we only have certain other forms of memory, such as implicit and/or procedural memory, from the trauma. The other group of theories is based on the idea that radically different types of memory are formed during trauma, and/or that some types of memory remain (for instance episodic memory) but take on a different form because of the shutting down of various functions. The theory of the zero process is of this second group. In order to discuss these ideas, we need first to describe the different forms of memory and their characteristics.

Recent decades have witnessed new discoveries by experimental psychologists and neuroscientists about the nature of memory functions. A key discovery has been the neural networks that underly the many different forms of memory. The complexity of memory can be seen by the fact that there are also a number of forms of short-term working memory (Schacter, 1996) based on transient brain changes. The various forms of longer-term memory are based on changes in brain microstructure— changes in the dendritic tree that grows out of one end of neurons that allow them to communicate with other neurons, and other changes in brain structure, including surely some of which we are at present unaware.

The conceptualization of different forms of memory goes back a long way. The most famous case was a patient, known in the literature as H.M., who had both left and right sides of his hippocampus removed, as part of surgery to control intractable epilepsy, in the 1950s (Schacter, 1996). With the loss of this key structure in the limbic system, H.M. lost the ability to form new memories. He could remember his past before the surgery well enough but if he met a doctor, and the doctor came back the next day, H.M. would not recognize him, having no memory of the previous meeting. At least, he had no perceptual memory, or what is called explicit or episodic memory. This is what people usually mean when they use the term memory. But if the doctor had a tack in his hand that pricked H.M. when he shook his hand during the first meeting, then when he met the doctor the next day and the doctor stuck out his hand H.M. would pull his own back. When H.M. was asked why he had pulled back his hand, he made up an excuse, but clearly had no memory of the real reason. He could not remember the past meeting, nor the tack, but he also *could* remember—he had no episodic memory, but had an emotional or conditioned memory. H.M. could also retain memories of certain skills he learned but here too, the memory was not episodic—he could not "remember" the times he had learned and practiced but he got better at the task nonetheless, although his progress was slower than would be usual for someone with episodic memory abilities. This type of memory for skills is referred to as procedural memory, and is retained in the cerebellum, which is generally concerned with the coordination of movement. H.M. also was able to acquire knowledge, but more slowly because of the lack of episodic memory. This type of memory—knowledge memory—is referred to as semantic memory. H.M. also learned things such as the layout of a room, or about certain objects, slowly over time, a form of implicit memory. This type of memory is often confused in the psychoanalytic literature with procedural memory. It is a non-verbal, non-semantic, perceptual representation system which usually works in concert with the semantic memory system, but can be disconnected from it. These implicit memories involve areas in the temporal lobe, fusiform gyrus, and the occipital lobe for vision, but not the hippocampus. These seem to be areas that respond to the general shape and other properties of an object, not specific little details. These can be changed with experience without any conscious knowledge at the time or later, and with no explicit memory (Schacter, 1996, 2001).

To summarize the basic long-term memory systems known at present: we have episodic memory (which is what we usually mean when we use the term memory), procedural memory (related to motor patterns), emotional memory, semantic (knowledge) memory, and implicit perceptual memories. While separate systems, these different forms of memory usually work together. For instance learning a skill is slower for people like H.M. who lack the ability to form episodic (perceptual) memories, but eventually they can acquire the skill (procedural memory), even though they have no "memory" (meaning episodic memory) of having learned it. The semantic memory system has been shown to be linked to the perceptual memory systems, whether episodic or implicit. One further category worth mentioning is autobiographical memory, which involves an integration of various episodic memories and semantic memories into a narrative story of what happened in the past. As we will see, this distinction (between episodic and autobiographical memory), and a number of others mentioned and to be mentioned, are important in coming to an understanding of what actually happens to memory in trauma, and what post-traumatic memory consists of. Which is not to say that at this point anyone has all the answers in this area, but at least we know enough to know that some of the proposed ideas about post-traumatic memory are incorrect or incomplete, and we can point the way towards where better ideas may reside.

While psychoanalysis has much to learn from recent memory research, it also has some things that it can provide in terms of clarification. As psychoanalysts we know that all memories are to begin with unconscious, and only become conscious at times. But beyond this, we know that episodic memories are quite capable of being repressed and thus kept from consciousness. Thus the other name for episodic memories—explicit memories—is misleading. Shevrin (2002) presents research from his own lab and that done by others demonstrating that episodic memories can be, perhaps usually are, formed outside of consciousness. These unconscious episodic memories are not formed by amnesiacs with hippocampal damage. When they are formed they require some further mental actions in order to become conscious. This is a key piece of understanding that psychoanalysis can add to the present work on forms of memory. Quite a while ago Ernst Kris, in his classic study of repression and memory (1956b), took note of different kinds of memory when he pointed out that repression, for instance the powerful oedipal repression that happen at around age five, attacks largely autobiographical memory (built up of episodic memories), as well as the associated drives and affects. Motor skills (procedural memory), and knowledge (semantic memory) are left largely untouched. We could add to this that implicit perceptual memory is also not effected by repression.

At present many have proposed that what we call repression is only, or mainly, a product of memory changes, with the loss of episodic memories. In other words the episodic memories are not pushed into the unconscious but are rather simply done away with or never formed. When, after repression of an episode or conflict, we are influenced by unconscious memories of it (as Peggy was by her repressed sexual abuse), these are seen as implicit memories. This is misleading on many counts. Firstly, by equating episodic memories with explicit memories, there is the suggestion that they are always or usually conscious, and thus that when we are influenced by memories that we do not remember consciously, they must be implicit memories. Secondly, it ignores the fact that implicit memories are formed only slowly over time, and relate to general characteristics of a situation, objects, or people. Specific incidents, whether traumatic or important for other reasons, are retained through the formation of episodic memories. But, the argument continues by those who espouse the idea of a special class of implicit or unformed but influential memories, the precedence of implicit memories should be recognized at least during trauma, when the episodic memory network is knocked out of operation, and also during early infancy, when it has not yet developed. And, says a strong trend in this theory, when both of these things are present—early childhood and relational trauma—then you have not repression of episodic memories but survival of implicit, unrepresented states, therapy for which would involve not reconstruction and memory recovery, but reliving with the therapist.

When taken to an extreme—and this idea is too often, in my opinion, taken at least a bit too far—these conceptualizations negatively effect our ability to analyze not just traumas but other things as well. I do not want to be misunderstood. I am not saying that early infancy and infant caretaker interactions are not important, nor that certain forms of implicit, procedural, and affective memories from that time, and other times as well, are not retained and do not effect aspects of the way the person is in the world. My argument is, as I said, with the overextension of these views beyond their true explanatory range. (In order not to break the flow of the argument, I won't at this point discuss specific authors, of whom there are many, who present versions of this idea of unrepresented early traumas. Botella (2014) is a good example, while Hock (2014) and Scarfone (2014) present thoughtful counterarguments.) These views are often supported by ideas on memory and the timetable of the development of memory systems in infancy, including the idea that episodic or declarative memories can only be formed in later childhood, perhaps beginning at age two to three, and the idea that during trauma at later ages as well, episodic memory goes offline, and only other forms of memory are laid down.

The study of the memory capacities of infants has led to discoveries that have challenged many preconceptions. In a paper on trauma and memory during infancy, Coates (2016) reviews the research in this area and notes that it is now clear that there are memory capacities even in the womb, and that representational capacity is innate, with episodic memory by two months and intentionality by five months. It was previously believed that infants do not remember what happened to them before the maturation of the hippocampus at around 18 months, which is also when language is acquired. Before this only procedural, implicit, and emotional memory, which were there from birth, were proposed as operational. Partly this is because of a mistaken equation of both verbal and autobiographical memory with episodic memory. Verbal memory of course only functions with the acquisition of language, but episodic memory is only later tied to language. And language is not, even later, a necessary aspect of episodic memory. Autobiographical memory involves the integration of various episodic memories, verbal memories, as well as semantic (knowledge) memories, into a coherent narrative, or really sets of narratives, about the person's past. This is obviously a later acquisition, and is the type of memory most subject to distortion based on biases and defenses. But single episodic memories do not need language or a narrative, and it seems that episodic and procedural and implicit memories are all there in a primitive form at or soon after birth, and then develop over time. Perhaps some of the confusion has come about also because it is our episodic memory system that changes and grows the most through time, as language and knowledge and representational capacities develop, and the integration and coordination of various memories takes place. The implicit, emotional, and procedural memory systems mature somewhat in early childhood, but then are relatively unchanged through later life (Schacter, 1996, 2001).

How do these findings and ideas about memory relate to post-traumatic memory, and what further can we learn from our work with traumatized individuals? In Peggy's case, her memories of the sexual abuse by her mother, which took place between the ages of seven and eight, were intense little pieces of perception. There was the feel of her mother's body, the smell, and the feelings of disgust. As is the norm with this kind of memory, the feelings also behaved not like regular memories, but like immediate perceptions. This was more obvious in the sessions described involving the rape of Joyce at the start of this chapter, where the perceptual immediacy and intensity of the zero process was on full display. But Peggy also lived in two worlds, one of them dominated by a sense of disgust, fear, aloneness, and tension, which was a continuation into the present of her sexual abuse, as well as of the chronic situation of living with her mother. The idea that normal episodic memories are not formed during traumas such as Peggy experienced gains some support from the finding that during trauma, and during the remembering of trauma, the hippocampus has reduced functioning while the amygdala, another limbic system structure related to fear and emergency responses, is extremely active. Thus the idea has developed that a person during trauma is like H. M.: unable to consolidate long-term episodic memories because key structures, and especially the hippocampus, needed for this process are out of commission. All that would remain would be the implicit, procedural, and semantic memories that H.M. was capable of forming. This idea comes up against the clinical reality, however, that there are almost always at least some perceptual memories from severe trauma. We should remember that even with an immature hippocampus in infancy, there is good evidence for episodic memory. There is clearly some kind of disturbance in how these memories are laid down, and also in how they are processed over time, which I have described as aspects of the zero process, and which has some similarities to the episodic memories from very early in life. (Here we bump up against a huge topic, of the relation of the zero process to infancy, which I will leave on one side for now, and address in my next book, where I develop the idea of the **developmental zero process**.)

Thus there is something to the idea of hippocampal dysfunction and a disturbance in the process of forming episodic memories. It is just that this idea is taken too far when it is suggested that in trauma no episodic perceptual memories of any sort are formed. In fact, the memories that are formed are closer in their immediacy and experiential nature to perception than are regular episodic memories. What are also retained very powerfully are certain body feelings and actions either performed or that the person wished to perform and could not during the trauma. These could be taken as the survival of procedural memories from the trauma. But here again a better understanding the nature of procedural memory, which is formed from repetitively practiced and learned motor patterns, related to such things as walking, riding a bike, or using a fork and knife, would argue against this equation. The "body memories" from trauma are much more specific than the general motor patterns of procedural memories. For instance Peggy could feel the weight and heat of her mother's body against hers as she relived the abuse. These sorts of body memories are similar to the perceptual zero process memories, in that they have the character of very specific immediate lived experience. Peggy's body would tense up severely and she would at times close her eyes quite suddenly as we talked of these occurrences, and these actions were traced to specific bodily re-actions and actions from the abuse. The actions were specific and had the quality of immediate lived experience, either of motor actions or percep-tions of bodily states. Of course with repeated abuse episodes, some forms of both implicit memory and procedural memories are also formed, so that what emerged and influenced Peggy's life had contributions from all of these memory systems. But the therapeutic efficacy and importance of unearthing the pieces of episodic zero process memory argues that they are present, along with all the other usual suspects, in terms of memory sys-tems, when it comes to trauma and post-traumatic states.

Episodic memory goes through a number of changes and retranscrip-tions in the normal course of things. At the neurological level, it is first stored through the mediation of the hippocampus and medial prefrontal regions, the latter of which seem to be involved in the deep analysis of the input. Storage is at first in the temporal lobes, but over time the memories seem to be shifted and distributed to various areas in the cortex (Schacter, 1996). When one remembers, one actually reassembles the memory from these distributed pieces. With each reassembling, aspects of the memory are usually altered and connections to other memories made. Traumatic memories, such as Peggy's of her sexual abuse, or Joyce's of her rape, share in the perceptual quality and specificity of regular episodic memories, but they do not share the reworkings and retranscriptions. The memory fragments stay separate from the rest of the person's memories, and are never assembled together with other memories, episodic, semantic, and implicit, into autobiographical narratives. The fragments of the zero pro-cess memory are also separate from each other. Unlike more regular epi-sodic memories the pieces are not reassembled into a whole as they are remembered, but remain as bits and pieces. There does appear to be some sort of temporal sequencing when they are relived, as Joyce's reliving of her rape showed. Because of the lack of integration and retranscription, zero process perceptual memories change very little, if at all, over time. This is one of their greatest, and most consequential, differences from regular episodic memories.

It is telling, given the evidence for the reality of episodic memories from early childhood, how this evidence is often not assimilated. A demonstration of this resistance occurred when Gaensbauer and Jordan (2009) interviewed 30 therapists about their patients with early trauma. They reported that the therapists themselves tended to forget that they had patients with early trauma, for instance saying that they didn't until reviewing their charts, or at first remembering that they did, and then forgetting at a second interview until they were reminded again by the researcher. Gaensbauer (1994, 1995, also, Gaensbauer & Jordan, 2009) presents some of the most detailed examples of very early trauma. He notes that analysts have tended to see the effects of trauma, especially at young ages, as being through cumulative situations. On the other hand he notes that actual clinical reports show that even during the preverbal period children have very similar responses as adults to single incident traumas.

Gaensbauer's cases are instructive and riveting. A boy is taken to hospital at seven months because of an overdose while in the care of a babysitter, and at 21 months he plays in ways that show he remembers them cleaning up his vomit in the emergency room. At four in analysis, he plays in certain very specific ways, that show his memory of things from the early trauma, such as being taken by a fire truck. At age seven, he does not remember any of this, but he has an interest in emergency vehicles and has dressed up as a fireman for three years running for Halloween (Gaensbauer, 1995). A girl of nine months was in a serious car accident with her mother, in which the car went over a bridge and landed in a dry stream bed. The girl went from outgoing to retiring, lost weight, and had specific fears related to details of the accident, for instance absolutely refusing to sit in the back seat of her car, and getting restless in her highchair. In therapy with Gaensbauer (1995) at 22 months, the girl played out details of the accident that shocked the mother, who had herself been traumatized and had not discussed these details with her daughter. After the session there was an upsurge in symptoms. A girl who had seen her mother blown up by a letter bomb when one year old had PTSD (post-traumatic stress disorder) symptoms of reliving. "She appeared to experience frightening, intrusive imagery, both in nightmares and in daydreams. While Audrey had not been able to describe her nightmares in detail, her adoptive mother recalled that at three years of age she awoke crying and saying, 'It's messy all over!' while rubbing her head and neck. The next day she pointed to some bed sheets coloured with large burgundy spots and said to her mother, 'That's a bad dream.' Her mother responded that the spots looked like flowers. Audrey said, 'No, they're messy all over,' and moved her hand in front of her." (Gaensbauer, 1995, p. 132). In this case, the girl talked of details of the incident, such as her mother's limbs being blown off, of which she had never been told, and of which her adoptive mother wasn't certain, but that were confirmed by the original police report of the incident when it was consulted. The articles by Gaensbauer have many other similar examples, including the very detailed case report of a boy he treated who was attacked in the face by a dog when he was 21 months (Gaensbauer, 1994). I would urge readers interested in this issue to especially read this case report, and a similarly detailed one by Terr (2013), of a young girl abducted and traumatized at age 13 months.

One of the features demonstrated by these case reports is that post-traumatic perceptual memories remain largely unchanged from the preverbal period, in much the same manner as zero process memories of older children and adults. As the children mature, they are able to add verbal labels and more complex thought to these pieces of intense perception, which remain vivid and immediate. It is an interesting question to consider to what extent this happens when a child has received no therapy or other occasions to discuss their trauma. I have seen adult patients who have had specific traumas from one year of age or less, and I have been struck, as have many others, by the survival of very specific perceptual and body reactions from the early trauma into adulthood, and also by the helpfulness of analyzing by focusing on the details of the reactions and reconstructing what had actually happened. In these cases, reconstructing the trauma and connecting it to various physical and emotional reactions of the patients seemed to set something free, and we were then able to see and analyze how these fragments of unprocessed memory had become entangled with later conflicts and traumas and relational issues. I found that it was only once this was done that certain stubborn resistances and symptoms finally gave way to analysis, suggesting the importance of getting at these traumatic memories when they are present. (Space precludes my giving detailed case reports here, but I will do so in my next book, which will look in more detail into development, including very early development, and trauma.)

No discussion of trauma and memory would be complete without a mention of the issue of false memories and fabricated memories. Arguments related to this have played out especially powerfully in the popular press, where it has been predictably approached in a simplistic manner. While most researchers and clinicians have more nuanced views and clinical practices, the extremes often get the most attention. As an example, Brewin (2003), a memory researcher, describes how, when he and others in an advisory group gave a press conference in which they laid out a more balanced view of the recovered memory controversy, the journalists were frustrated, complaining that they had nothing to put in their headlines the next day. A good headline, but one unlikely to sell many papers, or get many hits in their electronic version, is that memory comes in many forms, is generally reliable, but also generally distorted at least in some of its details.

Brewin (2003) notes that those who discount repression and other forms of motivated forgetting, and argue for the ubiquity of false memory syndrome, play a game in which each study is looked at for its flaws, except the studies supporting their position, and since there are always flaws in studies, the studies of the opposite camp are discounted. He notes that it's the method the tobacco companies used in claiming that there was no definitive proof that smoking caused cancer. (Or, in a more recent example which has stymied efforts to deal with an unfolding global catastrophe, the same game played by deniers of climate change.) The burden of proof is always on the other side. Brewin suggests that one has to look more broadly at the phenomena that needs explaining and ask if the ideas of the skeptics themselves do the job of explanation, which he suggests they do not, while a more complex view of memory and forgetting and repression does.

Shevrin (2002, pp. 133–134) notes that "it is possible to distinguish between true and false memories objectively on the basis of brain and cognitive studies. Misinformation causing misreporting does not necessarily change the memory trace itself. Moreover, the memory trace of a real event is marked by sensory and perceptual features missing in the false memory report. It is also possible to train people so that they can distinguish true from false memories. There is one last consequential inference we can draw from these results: if others can detect true from false memories on the basis of a 'sensory signature,' or the presence of sensory experience, then so can the person possessing the memory. We can make discriminations among our own memories and we do so quite frequently; the intriguing question is why we fail to do so."

It is certainly possible to have false memories of abuse or other traumas. I have seen patients who have had these, or who have had family members who have had them, as have many clinicians. And, as described by Shevrin, they were often vague and lacked the sensory qualities of true memories, such as Peggy's memories of abuse, while at the same time being much more narratively elaborated, and usually insisted upon with certainty and clung to, rather than avoided and denied, as Peggy did with her memories. The fact that in these situations of false memory the person gets quite angry if the memories are questioned, suggests their use as a screen supporting repressions. Usually there is some kind of drive conflict or situations of neglect or other traumas, elaborated into a false memory of a trauma, which then serves to buttress the repression, thus suggesting one answer to Shevrin's question of why people fail to distinguish false from true memories—they do so when it serves purposes of defense against some other conflict or trauma. What is lacking in these false memories is not just the characteristic sensory intensity coupled with avoidance of true traumatic memories, but also the usual triggered reactions. In Peggy's case, in contrast, when she became sexually active she found she generally enjoyed sex, but reacted strongly if a man touched her genitals with his hand, as her mother had done. "I just couldn't stand it and wouldn't let them do it." This reaction was present from adolescence, and continued for many years during which the memories of the abuse were largely repressed and avoided.

False memories of trauma are just one type of a larger class of strong memories which are often mistaken for traumatic memories, but which are actually related to repressed drive conflicts and/or are screens for other issues and traumas. Another member of this class of memories are the so-called flash bulb memories of significant events. For instance most people, certainly in America, had this kind of intense memory of the moment when they heard that President Kennedy had been assassinated, while more recently people had similar intense memories of when they heard about the Challenger Space Shuttle explosion and about the attacks on the World Trade Centre in 2001. These types of memories are sometimes referred to when trauma and traumatic memories are discussed, even though they are not a product of trauma, in the sense of an ego shut down, and are not zero process memories, at least for most people (of course they could be for people who personally experienced the incident or who were close to people involved in the tragedies). These types of memories are presented as traumatic memories, and the fact that they are often not accurate, or are subject to later distortion, is held up as evidence that this is the case for traumatic memories. But, as Van der Kolk (2014) notes, while people's memory generally changes over time, prospective studies, for instance some that followed people long after they had fought in World War II, showed that their traumatic memories did not change.

In flashbulb memories we see a number of processes at work. Firstly, as the novelty of an occurrence increases, so does our arousal and retention of the details of the situation (Van Der Kolk, 2014). This is increased even more with high emotion, especially fear. Occurrences like the September 11 attacks are collective examples of this sort of a high fear, high novelty situation. At the same time these types of situations trigger past traumas for many people, and for almost all people they trigger universal fears and core conflicts, around abandonment as an example, or fears of attack and bodily injury. In this way, the memories of such occurrences come to serve as an expression of, and yet screen for, these universal fears and conflicts, as well as for individual ones.

Of course people also have individual occurrences of similar high novelty, high arousal situations, and these also can have the "flashbulb memory" intensity. Only when the arousal and fear go past a certain tipping point, and a traumatic process ensues, are true zero process memories formed. Trauma could be seen as an overshooting of an emotional arousal and memory system built by evolution to adaptively retain details of novel and dangerous situations. It can be very helpful for the memories of these sorts of situations to not simply be abstracted and integrated with others, but rather remain somewhat separate, and capable of rousing quick reactions when similar situations arise. But the overshoot leading to the formation of zero process memories is not adaptive, as the lack of integration and abstraction of the memories goes so far that reactions become overly literal and tied to details of the situation. An example of this would be how Peggy reacted to anyone touching her genitals, which interfered with her sex life. Because the memories from her mother were split off and some were repressed, she could not make use of them in an adaptive manner, for instance to become aware of when she was in danger or threatened from someone like her psychopathic husband. Zero process memories can also be used as screens. Cordelia's memory, of being told by her father about her mother's death seemed to both be a true traumatic memory, and to have been retained with some intensity because of its connection with oedipal and other repressed conflicts and, as we shall see, as a screen for the traumatic time that followed.

The fact that the memory is intense and bright and well retained only marks it as a screen memory—in other words, it has its intensity and strong retention on loan from the wishes, conflicts, and traumas that it screens. Whether it is also a traumatic memory or not has to be decided based on other criteria. Many traumatic memories do not behave like or look like classic flashbulb memories. And most flashbulb memories are not traumatic memories. Perhaps the confusion has come about for two reasons—because many traumatic memories are used as screens, and because even those that aren't do have an immediate intensity when they are relived. But this intensity has much more the character of a lived experience that cannot be controlled once it is set in motion, while the remembering of flashbulb memories does not have these qualities and, though intense, is more under the person's control, as is the remembering of other non zero process memories. In fact, in mixed situations such as Cordelia's memory of being told of her mother's death, her simply remembering the incident, even with a lot of the feelings of sadness and shock, was not enough for a positive therapeutic result. For this the incident had to be analyzed more deeply in two directions—towards the drive conflicts and traumas that it expressed and screened, and towards the more raw zero process memories embedded in the smoother narrative memory.

Having gone into some detail in relation to memories of single incident trauma, we are now well armed to approach the topic of chronic trauma. The term chronic trauma potentially covers a range of phenomena. We see all of these in Peggy's case. The term could simply refer to many traumas, following one upon another chronically. This situation certainly was present in Peggy's childhood. But, being as adaptive as we are, when situations are repeated, the child is not usually just passively traumatized again and again. Peggy ran away physically from a young age, staying as far away from her mother as she could. She also developed a lively fantasy life and intellectual interests as escapes. During chronic traumatization, there are also immediate responses. When someone knows that abuse is coming, they will usually go somewhere else in their mind, into fantasies, or picture themselves sitting in another part of the room, looking on.

There is another meaning of chronic trauma which overlaps with the one just discussed but is in certain respects different. In this meaning, chronic trauma would refer to chronic stresses caused by impingements and deprivations that do not rise to the level of true trauma, in the sense that they do not cause an ego shutdown and the formation of zero process memories, nor the adaptation of ongoing dissociation to protect against further traumatization. Kris (1956b) used the term strain trauma to refer to this type of trauma, distinguishing this from what he called shock trauma. It is one constituent of what is called developmental trauma or complex developmental trauma, which refers to the effects of ongoing trauma and neglect on a person. Van der Kolk (2014) puts forward the diagnosis of developmental trauma disorder, into which he and others have done extensive research. He notes that the symptoms are different from the classic PTSD symptoms of intrusive memories and hyperarousal. This diagnosis captures the all too common situation of ongoing traumatization and neglect in disruptive environments leading to multiple difficulties during development, and in adapting to adult life. Peggy is an example of this kind of problem. However, the now popular term developmental trauma encompasses a heterogeneous set of dynamics which are worth teasing out for both theoretical and clinical reasons. It includes shock trauma and the dissociations and other adaptations adopted in the face of continued shock traumas, as well as strain traumas and other forms of developmental interference such as deprivations, over gratifications, and psychological abuse.

Examples of strain trauma in Peggy's case would include her mother's strange behaviour and unpredictability. She described how her mother would be whispering and looking up at whoever she thought she was talking to, and then all of a sudden would lash out in a scary menacing voice at another imaginary figure. Peggy was always kept on edge by this sort of behaviour and tried to escape her mother's presence. Her mother would also walk around in see-through nightgowns throughout the day, sometimes wandering outside, mortifying Peggy. The dream of her pulling at her mother's leg, which led to emotional memories of doing that as a very young child, brought out quite poignantly the deprivation that Peggy had had to deal with throughout her childhood. Of course any of these situations of strain could, and I believe did at times, rise to the level of overwhelming trauma with the formation of persisting zero process memories. These we can unequivocally call traumas. However, I think it is confusing to designate strain and stress in general as versions of trauma, such as strain trauma, developmental trauma, or cumulative trauma. In these terms trauma is being stretched to include deleterious situations with different dynamics and effects. In relation to our topic of memory, they do not lead to the formation of those persisting forms of largely episodic memories mixed with semantic and traces of other forms of memory, with wide ranging effects, that I have called zero process memories. Rather, there are combinations of regular episodic memories, emotional memories, implicit memories, semantic memories, and the persisting effects are mediated either through direct effects on development and/or through various persisting defenses and adaptations related to the strain situations. An interesting aspect of ongoing developmental strain is something Kris (1956b) called the telescoping of memory, in which one memory is retained to stand for many many incidents which are collapsed into it. This telescoping certainly was present in Peggy's one retained emotional memory of tugging at her mother's leg, as her mother looked up, talking to the voices she was hearing. This captured what would most likely have been hundreds of incidents of various sorts with a similar configuration, in terms of Peggy's longing for her mother, and her mother's complete emotional absence, as she was lost in her hallucinated world.

One of the difficulties with the word trauma is that it is also a common non-technical term, and in this form it has a wide range of meanings, including designating something really really bad, and really really upsetting, that happens to someone. In this context to say something is not traumatic can easily be taken to mean that it wasn't so bad, and certainly not as bad as something else that one designates as a trauma. The problem with importing this use of the term into scientific theoretical thinking about trauma, is that we lose specificity and lose our ability not just to think clearly about, but also to see clearly, the various phenomena at play. Many things that are not traumatic in the narrower sense may have much worse effects than traumatic incidents. In the last chapter I presented the example of a patient who had a car accident which led to certain post-traumatic symptoms which lessened over a number of months. The effects of a trauma such as this are clearly as nothing compared to the effects of the deprivation suffered by Peggy in relation to her mother, even when these deprivations did not lead to a traumatic process. Making these differentiations between trauma and developmental interferences and environmental strain at the conceptual level allows us to ask questions about the interaction between the implicit, emotional, and telescoped memories from deprivation and other chronic developmental strains and interferences, and zero process memories from traumas, and to craft interventions appropriate for each situation.

Peggy lived in two worlds. This is not something that she had told anyone, or even fully articulated to herself, before her therapy. But she was very certain that this was how she had lived her whole remembered life. The part of her that few saw was alone, lonely, scared, and felt weak and helpless. These feelings carried forward into the present her feelings from living with her mother and later with her psychopathic and abusive husband. Much of the feeling content of this alternate reality came from the emotional and implicit and telescoped episodic memories from the deprivation and maltreatments in these two relationships that did not reach traumatic level. But the fact that these other realities continued on in this way, not just as strong or upsetting memories but as a living present—an alternate present—unintegrated with the rest of Peggy's present experience, owed much to the existence of zero process memories. These acted as an anchor that pulled the other memories into this alternative reality and held them there. This statement is an inference based on the finding that it is usually only when the zero process memories have been brought to light and the trauma constructed to some extent, are the various other conflicts and chronic developmental interferences that have become connected to the trauma able to be analyzed in a way such that they lose their hold on the person. This is something observed and reported on again and again by trauma therapists of various persuasions, although of course they do not use the terminology that I have introduced. (As an example, Phillips (1991) describes this with regard to his patient suffering from adult war trauma.)

What seems to happen is that when the core traumatic memories are constructed, the non-traumatic dynamics are no longer caught up in the other reality of the zero process. Once they are freed from this, they still need to be analyzed, and this can often be no easy matter. But at least there is now the possibility of their analysis. This is certainly not a one way street, and a single-minded concern only with reconstructing memories and reactions relating to traumas is not helpful. One needs a flexible technique which considers other connections when they come into focus—for instance the analysis of Cordelia's aggression and death wishes, and Oedipal conflicts, which had become entwined with her trauma, and in Peggy's case her neglect by her mother and husband, and the terrible feelings of loneliness related to this, and the repressed anger at her beloved father, to mention only a few examples. However, the opposite approach is also not helpful, and I bring up this technical issue here, at the risk of repeating myself, because ideas about the nature of early memory and of traumatic memory are often used to argue for a technique that stresses reliving in the transference, not just as one part of and one tool of therapy but as the whole of it and as the only tool, and as a replacement for memory recovery and construction of the reality of what happened. It is held by many that episodic memories are not available from early traumas, that it is especially these early developmental traumas related to deleterious caregiving that are causative of a whole range of problems, and that these early developmental traumas are encoded in implicit, non-representational memory, which can only be accessed through reliving in a new relationship with the therapist. I believe that there are problems with all of these ideas, and will be addressing a number of them further along in the book. I have tried in this section to address these ideas in their relation to different forms of memory.

While procedural and implicit memories are important in our general functioning, and in mental dynamics such as the automatization and proceduralization of coping strategies into unconscious defenses, as well as in preserving the general characteristics of early and later experience, episodic memories and their zero process versions play an important part in bringing about the effects of both chronic strain, developmental interference, and trauma. In the case of trauma, zero process memories do not lack representation, only verbal and narrative additions, as well as cohesion and integration with the rest of the person's memories. They include a specific form of perceptual, episodic memory, formed under the very special conditions of the traumatic process. Episodic memory, whether of the regular or post-traumatic variety, is functional almost from birth. I gave a number of examples of zero process perceptual memories from very early trauma described by child psychotherapists in order to make this point. Implicit memory, on the other hand, only stores the general qualities of objects. My feeling, based partly on experience with patients who have been in therapy or analysis previously, is that often the idea of unrepresented memory is used in situations where repression or dissociation of episodic memories is occurring. For instance we might have thought that Peggy's early experiences with her mother were stored only implicitly, in which case we might not have been as alert for the emergence of memories of tugging at her mother's nightgown while she was lost in a psychotic delusion, among many other perceptual memories from that time. Recovering these memories from dissociation and repression was not a mere intellectual exercise, as they were tied to powerful emotions related to the reality of what she had had to deal with.

Implicit and affective memories of the past situation were also important to understand and acknowledge and work with in Peggy's case. It is not a question of one or the other, but of giving each their due, and also to give their interaction its due. The discovery of the nature of different memory systems not based on immediate perception—emotional memory, procedural memory, implicit memory, semantic memory, and priming—has been an important addition to our knowledge. But they are not an explanation for every time, or even the majority of times, that we act or have a symptom and are not conscious of their causes.

Having travelled some distance down memory lane, trying to elucidate the true nature of traumatic memory, and arguing against using implicit memory or unrepresented experience as general explanations for post-traumatic effects, we now arrive at a place where we will need to explain such effects in more dynamic terms; terms related to the driven nature of zero process memories, and the various defensive maneuvers that attempt to keep these memories from our awareness. These explanations are the topic of the next chapter.

Chapter 3

The Zero Process Drive and Zero Process Defenses

The Zero Process Drive

One of the most striking characteristics of zero process memories is the push for them to be actualized as an immediate present experience. I have called this—one of the defining characteristics of the zero process— the zero process drive. All true zero process memories possess and are animated by this push. I designated it as a drive because I think there is evidence that it is an independent motivational center. This is especially manifest in the behaviour of zero process internal objects (introjects), as was discussed in the last chapter, and in the alters of dissociative identity disorder, to be discussed at the end of this chapter. The sexual drive could serve as an example of a functional drive: at any time there will be a push to actualize certain wishes, and something needs to be done with this push: either action to fulfill the wishes, repression, redirection, sublimation, or combinations of these. The sexual drive as such goes through processes of development over time—for instance Cordelia was moving into her oedipal phase, which involves childhood genital sensations and wishes, at the time of her trauma. There is an inherent developmental push to this unfolding of the developmental timetable of sexuality, but this is quite a different type of push or drive than the functional drive of the sexual impulses at any given moment in time. We may ask, though, how zero process memories come to have characteristics similar to the sexual and aggressive drives? I have suggested that the ego breakdown during trauma means that the regular sequence of the construction of present experience and its memorialization is stopped short, and that there is a normal push to complete this sequence.

Regular memories may be evoked by a situation, but once evoked we have reasonable control over them, being able to scan them back and forth or put them aside. The very different situation with zero process memories is illustrated by the descriptions of General Romeo Dallaire (2016), U.N. forces commander and witness to the Rwandan genocide he was helpless to stop, as no country or the U.N. responded to his pleas for

DOI: 10.4324/9781003283218-4

military support. He describes being back in Canada for years, trying to drown out with work the insistent memories of the horrors he had witnessed and the helplessness he had experienced. "And so I worked. For months and years I worked and worked. And nothing disappeared, except the arm pain. My thoughts, my memories—everything I'd experienced in Rwanda—remained digitally clear, and kept playing out in slow motion in front of my eyes, like a teleprompter" (p. 26). No matter how he tried, the memories came. And they did not come as memories but as perceptions, even more clear than regular perceptions. It is this push toward intense and repetitive living out as an immediate experience that is the zero process drive. Again, Dallaire's words say it better than mine: "Those first two years back, I could not divorce myself from Rwanda. I'm not even sure I could say the war was over; I was still living it. I kept two huge filing cabinets, full of notes, cables, documents, and photos, beside my bed. Locked inside, I had the whole genocide. The presence of those files was like something alive, pulsing in the corner, waiting to strike" (2016, p. 52). A filing cabinet of powerful, pulsing experiences, waiting to strike. That is the zero process drive.

While it may at first seem that the memories impose themselves unopposed on the person, a closer look suggests that this is rarely the case. Dallaire could never refuse an invitation to talk about the genocide. This gave him somewhere to put the memories or, more accurately, realities that kept intruding. He describes how during talks he would hold up a watermelon and cut it with a machete, demonstrating what was done to the heads of victims. He induced in his audience at least a little bit of the horror that he was experiencing. This was somewhere else that he could put these things. So while the zero process pushed, Dallaire pushed back. What resulted was some kind of a compromise between the drive to recreate the past, and opposing forces. Talking about these events and inducing the feelings in others by cutting the watermelon was an active process and to some extent a reversal of the helplessness he had felt. Dallaire describes how he was asked to testify at the trial in Tanzania of a number of the perpetrators of the genocide. He was urged not to go by people in the U.N. because of safety concerns—there were death threats against the General who couldn't stop telling the story of what had happened. He was urged not to go by his psychiatrist and others who were concerned for his mental health. But as he explained it, he could say nothing but yes to anything to do with the genocide. "I was pushed by a driving force that overrode logic, the demands of my health, even my fears that I'd fail again. It kept pushing me forward but I did not understand it" (2016, p. 86). What Dallaire describes is another compromise, a type of sublimation similar to the sublimation of sexual drives. Many of our passions, the things that we cannot not do, as so eloquently described by Dallaire, are sublimations of zero process drives.

But these compromise formations, defenses, and sublimations look different from those related to the sexual and aggressive drives. They are more closely tied to specific concrete memories. This is explained by the differences between zero process drives and id drives. The drives of the id are much more malleable. In fact, this is one of the key discoveries made by Freud about the nature of such drives. His libido theory posited not just that there was a sexual drive but that the energy of this drive was much less tied to specific sexual wishes, acts, or objects than had previously been believed. The energy that came in the end to power adult sexuality was conceptualized by Freud (1905) as beginning as an investment in pleasure and the various bodily areas and people that produced it. This energy, or libido as Freud came to call it, could be displaced from one thing onto another, it could be inhibited and held back in its aim, and it could be fused with the aggressive drive, to form such things as sadism. Later other authors (most importantly Hartmann, 1955; Jacobson, 1964; and Kris, 1955) distinguished neutralization of a drive, in which its aims are changed, muted, or become more distant from the original, from displacement and fusion. If a young boy wants to kill his father but gleefully crushes insects instead, we have displacement with little neutralization or fusion. If he teases his father, we can see fusion of the aggression with fond and loving feelings at work, while he may tease his dog, demonstrating fusion and displacement. If he were to try to better his father by knowing more than him about some topic, we can see neutralization of the original death wishes at work, with little fusion or displacement. I touched on these ideas about drive energy and its transformations when discussing repression, which I believe uses partially neutralized aggressive energy to block the conscious awareness of such things as forbidden wishes and traumatic memories.

Aggression in general, in partially neutralized form, performs not only useful but essential tasks, in setting up boundaries and structures within the mind. A good ability to neutralize aggression is related to resilience, while deficits in neutralization lead to deficient or unstable structures— such as those set up by repressions and self/other differentiation—and thus to psychological fragility. I will discuss this aspect of drive neutralization in chapter four, on borderline disorders. I realize that these ideas about energy transformations have been rejected by many theorists and theories of psychoanalysis. Other understandings of relationships, for instance based on a basic mammalian instinct of attachment, are on the ascendance. I myself think that Freud's drive and energic theories are both valid and extraordinarily useful, and that we have lost an important conceptual tool with their downfall. I propose to demonstrate their usefulness in this book largely by using them, with some discussion of theory. In my next book, in discussing normal development and the normal construction of reality, including in scientific theories, I will present a deeper theoretical set of arguments in favour of energic ideas in psychoanalysis.

To continue with the comparison of zero process drive versus id drives: the most striking difference between the two is that the id drive is not only highly malleable, being capable of fusion and neutralization, but that it is not tied to specific memories or objects. Or at least this tie is not obligatory. Of course early investments of the libido are hard to let go of, but this is still a long way from the tight and indissoluble lock between the push of a zero process drive, and its object. Dallaire could only relive exactly the same sights and sounds and smells that he had experienced as the genocide unfolded. This is not to say that there could not be some amount of displacement—from a person's head to a watermelon, and from Dallaire witnessing the scene to members of his audience witnessing it. But the specificity of zero process memory fragments always exerts a strong pull, and the sublimations of people's zero process drives never stray very far from home. Cordelia would react whenever anyone was sick with quick action (something she had not been able to do with her mother), with alternatives to traditional medical treatments (which had proved unable to save her mother), with caring but also often with frustration and anger that the person was not taking enough action on their own behalf (which proved to be related to the anger she felt at her mother for abandoning her by dying). Cordelia was passionate about finding cures and investigating different forms of treatment. But the stark reality of what had happened to her mother was always close at hand, as shown by the clinical material near the beginning of this book. This can be compared to sublimations of id drives. The anal wish from early childhood to mess and play with and smell faeces, and the pleasure taken in all of this, can be sublimated into a pleasure in cleaning up things—for instance the messy pile of ideas and thoughts in a book on the theory of trauma—and structuring them and making them come out nice and clean and neat, but perhaps not too neat, in order that they not be too boring, but still have some of the zing of the original anal pleasures. The energy and interest in this task can still be connected to the anal wishes even as the task moves quite far away from the original. The original is there in the deeper unconscious but does not intrude into the sublimated task to the same extent as when the sublimation of a zero process drive is involved.

Given these differences, why call the push of the zero process a drive at all? Here, for all their differences, we come up against the major similarity between the primary process drives and the zero process drive: they exert a continuous push towards expression. In this, both these types of drives differ from affects such as anxiety, sadness, or anger. These usually are roused by a specific situation, whether an external one or something internal, and then of course they exert a push for expression. But once they gain expression, there is no further push—unless the affect is connected to an id drive or a zero process memory and its drive. This continuous push for expression in the case of zero process drives means that dynamics involving them stay with people throughout their lives, and have a stability and persistence. There are zero process drive/defense conflicts and dynamics, just as there are the better-studied id drive/defense dynamics. The strong pull towards repeating aspects of the trauma is based on these. Or to be more accurate, the push to complete repetition is based on the zero process drive itself, while what actually happens, which is a compromise between repetition and its avoidance, is a product of the push of the zero process drive to recreate the trauma, and the defenses that oppose it.

We now turn to a consideration of the defenses used in relation to trauma and the zero process drive. In the last section of chapter one, on overwhelming from outside versus overwhelming from inside, I outlined the theory of defenses presented in my previous book (2009, see also 2013a). I will in the discussions to follow be using the basic distinction introduced there, between counterforce defenses used against drives, and attentional defenses used against unpleasant realities, in investigating the nature of zero process defenses and zero process dynamics. I have tried to explain aspects of the theory as I use it, but if the reader finds things to be unclear, I would suggest referring to the last part of chapter one, or to the glossary at the back of this book.

Repression

Psychoanalysts have repeatedly asserted that because post-traumatic memories are not properly formed or have not become fully representational, they cannot be repressed as other memories can be. They are rather dealt with by dissociation and similar defenses. On the other hand, it is easy enough to observe clinically that traumatic memories are in fact often repressed. Peggy's repression of memories of her mother's sexual abuse of her between ages seven and eight is an example of this not uncommon phenomenon. How to reconcile the assertions with the clinical realities? One needs to divide up the post-traumatic memories into their drive component (zero process drive), which is definitely dealt with by counterforce defenses such as repression, reaction formation, and splitting of the identity, and the memory component that acts like a present reality, which is dealt with by denial defenses and special zero process defenses including dissociation. The assertion that one cannot repress post-traumatic memories is partially correct for the "behaves like a present experience" component, but not for the drive component.

Repression is not an "experience near" action of the ego. It takes place silently with reference to consciousness. We know it first from its effects—something disappears from consciousness. There is no awareness that it is lost, and yet there is a resistance if we try to bring it back to the person's attention. As psychoanalysts have turned their attention to other defenses, especially to splitting and projective identification, repression has faded from view. Some analysts claim that repression has literally faded from view—that it is a defense that is used much less often now than in previous times, either because earlier times were more "repressed," or because we now see more ill patients who use splitting and projective identification.

In discussing this, it is helpful to go back to basics. A defense is an inference. We can observe some surface manifestations which may give us a clue that a defense is present, such as for instance that someone has no memories for a period in their life or, in Peggy's case, that she had not remembered the sexual abuse by her mother, and then some memories returned. But *we infer the actual mechanism of the defense from the nature of the resistance we meet as we attempt to approach certain memories, feelings, etc.*

Peggy would talk about the sexual abuse for a few minutes, but would then put her hands over her face, and change the topic. The avoidance was quite plain, as was the motive for the defense, as she shuddered and seemed fearful and disgusted. When she talked about her mother being in her own world and often not paying attention to her, I asked her if she did pay attention sometimes. Peggy said she did or must have, but when pushed to actually come up with an instance, she fell back on generalities. When I pointed this out, she said that her mother would sometimes hold her close and pet her, like a doll. She then realized that this did not feel good either, and that her mother was treating her as a thing. Her constant attempts to shift her attention to general comments like "she must have paid attention to me sometimes" demonstrate the workings of her denial of the full extent of her mother's lack of contact with her. One thing this also demonstrates is that it is often as one interprets what one intuits is being unconsciously hidden, that the structure of the resistance, and thus of the defense, can be seen. And then if one further confronts or interprets the resistances, such as my pointing out that Peggy seemed to be clinging to the idea of her mother as connected to her, then the response to the interpretation clarifies further the dynamics of the defense. For instance, Peggy trying to still find ways in which, or instances where, her mother was connected to her or loving, demonstrated further the attentional nature of her denial defense against the reality of her mother's psychotic state, as Peggy tried desperately to construct an image of at least some normal interactions.

Attentional defenses such as those used by Peggy are ego actions with which we are generally familiar, and thus we can easily relate to them, and in fact what people often find hard to understand is that the person using this mechanism is quite unaware of it. The situation is somewhat different in the case of repression. Everyone is familiar with at times making strenuous efforts to suppress an impulse, bad memory, or feeling, and with what it feels like to try to push these things away from conscious awareness. Yet when we lose all conscious access to a set of memories and feelings for an extended period of time, there seems something uncanny about the process. I would contend that this is because the mechanism of repression involves drive transformations that are quite far from the sort of things that can become conscious. We usually only become conscious of perceptions and some inner feeling states. Even thoughts can only become conscious through connections to perceptions, of words heard or images or words that are seen.

The transformation of aggression into a force that opposes the forward movement of an id or zero process drive is the sort of mechanism that has few perceptual or affective referents, and thus little access to consciousness. We infer the inner workings of this mechanism from an important but easy to misconstrue set of reactions that occur as we attempt to analyze repression. People have a burst of anger when their repressions are challenged. We might think of this merely as a reaction of repudiation which one would expect whenever a person is faced with an unwelcome reality, with no deeper significance. However, it differs from many other common instances of irritation and fending off of unwelcome truths. As an example, Peggy was certainly none too pleased to talk of her mother's lack of interest in her, and her strange and embarrassing behaviour. She would voice her disinclination to talk of this, sometimes saying, "that's enough!" However, if I brought up the sexual abuse in relation to something else she had been talking about, or even if she did this, and then I pursued it and asked her for associations, Peggy would have a flash of anger, and give me an angry look, which was quite out of keeping with her usual friendly attitude. Once, when the conversation had gone on even longer than usual on this topic, Peggy came back to the next session telling me, "you know, I was really angry at you after last session, and I stayed angry." She said this with some emotion, and seemed a bit surprised at how she had sustained her anger.

Now, such a response may seem a very slender thread indeed on which to hang an assertion about the deeper mechanism of repression. But it does not hang from a few threads but from a thick rope, made up of thousands of observations of different aspects of resistance, as well as other observations related to childhood development. One important set of observations are similar to what I just described: comparisons of responses by the same patient to analysis of different defenses. Here many of the complex interlinked variables can be kept relatively constant, allowing a comparison of the specific reactions we want to explore. In a longer psychotherapy or psychoanalysis, one can also observe the way these reactions change over time. In general, when one confronts a denial or dissociative defense, one gets resistance and an amount of irritation or anger which seems commensurate with our bringing things to awareness which are bound to cause pain. In the case of repression one either gets nothing—a blank mind—or denial and other resistances of secondary defenses or, especially as the exploration proceeds, one gets a burst of anger that comes rather suddenly and surprises the analyst and often the patient as well.

As the analysis of the repressed conflict or trauma proceeds, this anger often organizes itself into a specific type of negative transference usefully designated as a transference resistance. This is what happened as we pushed deeper into Peggy's repressed blaming of her father for not protecting her from her mother, and into her zero process memory fragments from her sexual abuse by her mother. She became reluctant to come, and tried to change the topic to nicer things when she did, which was a transference of her avoidance of being in the house with her alternately embarrassing and scary mother, and then trying to make the world at home seem nicer and not so scary through fantasy and her more positive interactions with her father. She would sometimes put her hands over her face and peek out between her fingers, as she might have done when dealing with her mother's strange behaviour. There is much that could be discussed about this transference, including its many layers and the countertransference responses on my part, but in relation to the topic at hand, I would point out that the change of the repression first to an immediate aggressive reaction upon confrontation, and then to this complex resistance, is also a sign of the malleability of the aggressive drive. This transmutation of the original angry response into sustained transference resistances is another of the pieces of evidence, another of the threads in the rope of evidence, for the derivation of repression from partially transformed aggressive drive energy.

Freud described the transference resistance in his papers on technique (Freud, 1912, 1915), noting that as one analyzed the patient's repressions, eventually some part of the transference that served well to block the further progress of the analysis would get pushed to the fore and become most prominent. He noted that this did not mean this was the most important aspect of the patient's past relationships, but rather that it owed its prominence to its usefulness as a resistance. Freud suggested it was important not just to trace this transference to its roots, but also to point out the resistive function that it was serving. This well-known aspect of classical Freudian technique has fallen into disuse (and in some quarters, disrepute) with the rise of object relations and relational theories and techniques, but it contains an important insight into the nature of repression, which was not conceptualized by Freud. The transference resistance only becomes fully theoretically comprehensible once we conceptualize repression as formed from malleable aggressive drive energy, and understand this resistance as the interpersonal expression of it. In the burst of anger when repression is starting to break down, we see an intrapsychic defense explode out into the interpersonal sphere, and in the transference resistance we see this explosion become more organized and stabilized into an interpersonal relationship. (And we will see in discussing projective identification in chapter four, on borderline disorders, that this too is actually a version of this same explosion of an intrapsychic counterforce into the interpersonal sphere, but without much subsequent modulation.)

Even though repression as an intrapsychic phenomenon is experience distant and difficult to picture, it can be transformed into the phenomenon of the transference resistance, and brought into the interpersonal sphere. Thus this most enigmatic of defenses becomes, if handled correctly, eminently analyzable. It is through this transformation of a major intrapsychic structure into a type of transference resistance that in favourable situations is analyzable, that psychoanalysis can bring about structural change. Freud and the early analysts studied how this could be done in the case of drive/defense conflicts related to the id or primary process. I would argue that if one wishes to bring about structural change in relation to the hold traumas have on the lives of people, one needs in the same manner to analyze zero process drive/defense conflicts, which in the case of trauma involves repression and splitting of the identity. I will describe splitting of identity as the prototypical zero process counterforce defense at the end of this chapter, and will consider specific techniques for the analysis of this defense in chapter five. Here we will proceed with repression.

Let me now present in outline an example of what I mean by repression being used against a zero process drive. I described the moment when Cordelia was told by her father that her mother would not be coming back, and some of the reactions she had at the time, including the feeling of a black hole invading her. Despite remembering this moment of trauma reasonably well, she had very little sense for what happened in the months that followed. She knew she had not been taken to the funeral. She thought she knew this because she had been told. She had a memory of sleeping beside her father in bed, which had significance related to a number of dynamics. Of course she was very young, only four, and yet the more we talked about the issues around her mother's death the more often Cordelia was struck by how there was a true blank spot in her mind for the time after the fateful dinner, even as she remembered the dinner and her father's words and her responses quite well. We had talked about this time often, in terms of how her usually loving grandparents and her father were quite distant and unavailable as they were consumed with grief at her mother's death at such a young age. It made sense that this situation exacerbated Cordelia's feelings of having been abandoned.

Later in the therapy, as I interpreted Cordelia's temporal shifting of her trauma (a defense to be described later), in which her trauma lived not in her past but in her future, not as a memory but as a fear, feelings of desolation and being alone emerged more strongly than previously, including in the transference. We realized, and she started to remember, that she was invaded by these overwhelming feelings for the weeks and months after her mother's death. As we talked, two memories popped up during different sessions, both involving a babysitter – a teenager from the neighbourhood. In one of these memories, the babysitter jumped out from hiding and made a funny face, leading to her and Cordelia breaking out into gales of laughter. "I think I remember it because I broke out of my feelings of desolation and actually smiled and laughed. Otherwise, I was just sullen. There's a picture of me with my grandparents—maybe I should bring it in—where I just look so miserable." The second memory was of watching this babysitter talk to a neighbourhood boy. They seemed to be flirting in a way which felt warm and friendly to Cordelia. "It was full of life and excitement and possibility," she said. Both she and I wondered if here too the memory was remembered because it countered a sense of lifelessness and lack of a future that Cordelia had felt at that time. And finally, there was a memory that Cordelia had always remembered very well, and had recounted near the beginning of her therapy, in which she is so excited that she cannot sleep, because her father has told her that a young woman was going to be coming to stay and take care of them. She was to be a live-in nanny, although Cordelia thought of her already, as she remembers it, as a replacement mother, or almost as her mother come back in another form. Her father did end up marrying this woman years later, but Cordelia was sorely disappointed from the start in her hopes, as the woman turned out to be quite rigid and harsh with her.

As the analysis of the period just after her mother's death deepened it became clear why Cordelia had always retained such detailed memories of being told by her father that her mother was not going to come back, and of the end of this period when she got excited about the nanny coming. Her father had said that they had to stick together as a family, and he had the youngest child on his lap. They were all together in this memory, and the dark black hole was only beginning to invade her and take her over. This was the start of everything. The conversion symptoms related to Cordelia's stomach being full, and loss of appetite, and stomach pains, seemed to come from this incident. The two incidents with the babysitter that popped up as we were talking of this period were screen memories, as was the memory of being told about her mother's not coming back. Calling something a screen memory may be seen as saying that it is an unimportant incident, or even a made up one, hiding the real thing. But in reality a screen memory is what is left once repression has done its work. It is a compromise between the repressing forces and the attachment to the memories. Kris (1956b) suggested that while aggression is used to set up the repression barrier, the libido that has been partially withdrawn from the repressed memories invests the screens, giving them that feeling of intensity and specialness that they carry ever after.

Each of the screens in this situation stressed aspects that were the opposite of the trauma that was repressed: people being around, fun, happiness, and perhaps most of all, aliveness and a future. But they also contained the ideas of loss, both directly and because even as she remembered them, especially the two incidents with the babysitter, Cordelia could feel the desolation at the edge of the memories. These two memories also were screens for instinctual (primary process) drive conflicts, for instance her memory of the babysitter flirting screened Oedipal fantasies and wishes. In fact, in Cordelia's case the repression of these wishes proceeded in tandem with the repression of her trauma. The babysitter memories were relatively everyday memories used as screens, while the memory of being told of her mother's death was a shock trauma, and the start of a longer period of trauma. The first part of a trauma, and other shocking events after that, are often heightened in memory and used as a screen for the repressed portions of the trauma. This is an almost universal dynamic with important implications for clinical technique.

The feelings from the months after the fateful dinner might seem, and certainly would have been, feelings both related to the loss of Cordelia's mother and the loss of her grandparents and father as they were in deep mourning. But I would argue, based on what came before and after, that something else was also going on, somewhat masked by the more straightforward reactions. I would argue that Cordelia was demonstrating the aftermath of a trauma, in which the zero process drive led to repeated shocks of the feeling of complete abandonment that she had felt at the moment of being told of her mother's death. These, and the memories and thoughts attached to them, were then repressed. I would present as evidence for this the fact that as I interpreted what was going on during this time after the trauma, there was the burst of irritation that I described as characteristic of the weakening of a repression, and later its moulding into a mild but characteristic transference resistance. As this was uncovered through the analysis of the screen memories and worked through, and the repression of the zero process memories that kept intruding at that time, and that played out throughout her life, were partially undone, there was a change in certain anxieties and symptoms. There was also a deeper integrative understanding of how this fitted in with all the other things that were going on in her young life at the time, as well as how it manifested later, for instance in Cordelia's adolescence as she tried to deal with this terror of abandonment, and in her adult life as she was beset by it, without knowing why, about four years into each relationship. She connected empathically and more deeply with the little abandoned girl of that time, after her mother had died. There was a back and forth between resistance, where Cordelia found reasons not to come, and then insights into all sorts of connections to later times where the repressed zero process drives returned in adulthood and shaped her adult life.

To return to the original traumatic period: there are of course many things going on in the mind at any one time, especially in the mind of a four-year- old with so much to deal with and so much growing up to do. But one of the important things going on was, I think, that at first the zero process drive kept playing out bits of the trauma, and that then repression stepped in and partially held this process at bay. In a girl with good ego functioning such as Cordelia, a main defense is selective repression that, as in the case of id drives, specifically targets the drive and what is associated with it. (Selective repression will be discussed in more detail in chapter four, in the section "Repression, Internalization, and Trauma.") This is not the end of the matter in the aftermath of trauma, any more than it is the end of the matter when id drives are repressed. I described how Cordelia projected her aggression, and became scared of intruders, as an example of secondary defenses, even though the core of her death wishes were repressed. Similarly, Cordelia would throughout her life have to use various auxiliary defenses to help out her repression of the zero process push towards repetition. Some of these secondary defenses, including avoidance, were described when I first presented some material from her therapy. I will discuss these non-repressive defenses in more detail in the next two sections.

Some readers may feel that what was actually happening was that I was enacting the emotional withdrawal of Cordelia's caretakers after her mother's death by interpreting the trauma rather than empathizing with her lived experience of the time, and thus she relived an anger at me for that. This is possible, but in fact we had for quite a while looked at this period from this angle, trying to get in touch with what it must have been like, but with the whole process seeming somewhat abstract and intellectual, until Cordelia herself started noticing the strange blank space in her mind and life, and we inquired into it. I did of course then interpret the repetition of the traumatic abandonment, and met with some resistance, which I pointed out to her. This is also the point at which some may think I was enacting the abandonment, and there may well be truth to this idea. But it does not preclude the aggression from being also a resistance related to the breaking down of a repression. Only the further course of the therapy, including shifts in transferences and symptoms and resistances and integrations over time, would let us decide. All these shifts took place in Cordelia's case, and made it evident that she had partially repressed the push to repeat. For all of our work previously, which had led to very heartfelt sadness, it was only as we analyzed her feelings and repressions from this shadowy time of the months after the trauma, that there were marked changes in Cordelia's symptoms. She gained weight. She also was not as scared or triggered when there was something suggestive of abandonment, and did not feel as strong a pull to constantly save people. She said with a laugh that now she could delegate it, giving them advice about who else they could seek help from. These did not disappear all at once or completely, but slowly over time the pull towards repetition lessened. This had nothing to do with us working directly on the particular symptom, such as not eating and weight loss, as we did not discuss them much during this stretch of time when we worked on the repression. The pull did not disappear, and it probably never does disappear in cases of major trauma. But we can see how when the pull is less, this allows a kind of sublimation of the zero process drive towards repetition, with more flexibility in what one does with it—for instance taking an interest in people's health but not having to save them in a panicky way.

Some readers may argue that the improvement was a product of a transference. I would agree with the argument, but would take it further: just as when one penetrates to a repressed instinctual drive conflict, the conflict tends to be transferred into the analysis, so too does this happen with zero process drive conflicts. The repetition now happens to a greater extent within the therapy and with the therapist. The extreme of this can be seen in Joyce's reactions that I described, where she relived one part of her trauma as if it were an immediate experience, with me as her abuser. So also with Cordelia there was definitely an aspect of transference cure – a cure based on the displacement of conflicts related to the trauma into the analysis. This by itself is not a sign of failure, just a stage in therapy, well enough known in the analysis of drive/defense conflicts. Cordelia's external symptoms increased and decreased based partly on the trans-ference dynamics. As we were well into the analysis of the repressed period after her mother's death, she at times got worse, lost many of her gains, and kept wanting to cancel appointments. I interpreted the avoidance and fear of the intense emotions from the loss of her mother, and more memories and feelings bubbled up. She had bouts of extreme anxiety, and feeling like she was barely alive. She said she felt "de-animated." She became convinced that this feeling of de-animation and deadness was what had overcome her in the months after her mother's death—the months that until recently had been a blank space in her conscious mind.

This was a long but very productive phase of working through the insights. If we look more closely we can see what one part of the deeper dynamics of working through are, and even why we need this working through process for change to stabilize—or, to put it differently, for true structural change to happen. Cordelia was not as unfailingly friendly to me and positive about the therapy during this phase of working through. She would at times be irritated or negative, but we worked in the face of this attitude and moved towards some of the deepest insights of her therapy. Kris (1956a) noted in his classic description of what he called the "good hour," that such an hour often starts seemingly inauspiciously, with the patient resistant and irritable, which he regarded as a sign of the weakening of defenses—I would say specifically that it represents the aggression set free as the repressive counterforce which was formed by the aggression starts to crumble. It is only the working through process that allows this aggression, formerly structured into a repression, to find other uses, and for the repressive structure to be permanently modified. As examples of other uses of the aggression, Cordelia's sense of self and identity became much firmer and more boundaried, and she was able to push through more forcefully on certain plans she formed related to deep interests of hers.

What is commonly referred to or diagnosed as post-traumatic stress disorder is the playing out of the zero process drive without enough selective repression to at least partially control the repetition in dreams and in waking life. If repression, and other counterforce defenses such as compartmentalization and splitting of the identity, can be brought to bear in a significant manner on the zero process drives left in the aftermath of a trauma, then the symptoms and repetitions will look less and less like what we associate with classic PTSD. The drive will be tamed, in a manner of speaking. Zero process memories as flashbacks will be triggered less often and less intensely; the appearance of the trauma in dreams will be more disguised; repetitions also will be less common and more subtle; and various symptoms such as phobias and conversion symptoms will be more stable and serve as containers for the trauma, which will not flood the person's life to the same extent. In these situations, as I described with Cordelia and Peggy and Joyce, the trauma repetition and alternate zero process reality is everywhere in the person's life, but is kept in check enough, that often the extent of its invasion of the person's life only becomes clear as attention is paid to it in therapy.

The immediate aftermath of any trauma will involve repetitions in dreams and waking life, and look much like PTSD. But from this point things can go in a number of directions, and in each direction to a variable extent. If the trauma is not too extreme, the repetitions may serve as part of the normal healing process in a bland trauma, and over a number of months the zero process memories will be converted into more regular memories. If selective repression and other counterforce defenses manage to work sufficiently against the push towards repetition, one gets the sorts of situations I have described in general terms just above, and illustrated concretely in the cases of Peggy and Cordelia. If counterforce defenses cannot hold the zero process push to repetition in check because of the severity and/or continuing nature of the trauma, or because of certain ego weaknesses, one gets something approaching what is described as PTSD, which Romeo Dallaire's descriptions of what he went through after coming home from Rwanda capture so well.

Dissociation

Dissociation is the defensive maneuver associated most closely in people's minds with trauma. The early investigators of trauma, most notably Janet, explained the effects of trauma through noting that it caused a dissociation, in the sense of a set of memories that were cut off from association with the other memories, feelings, and thoughts of the person, so that they could not be worked over and thus the feelings and impulses connected with them could not be abreacted. Breuer (Breuer & Freud, 1895) described essentially the same situation, using the term hypnoid states. The revival of interest in trauma over the last decades has been accompanied by a similar revival with respect to dissociation. This has happened within psychiatry and psychology, and also within psychoanalysis. There has been an unfortunate tendency for many taking part in this revival to take an either/or attitude regarding the importance, or even the existence, of repression versus dissociation. It is interesting that this plays out the same attitude, in reverse, from the early days of psychoanalysis, where Freud (1910, 1914) insisted that what Breuer and others saw as dissociation was really a product of defensive maneuvers related to repression. One of my aims in this book has been to follow those (for instance Ira Brenner, 2001, 2004, 2014) who try to go against these trends, by holding onto insights about the workings of repression and of dissociation, and not reducing either one to the other. By doing this we gain a better and more differentiated understanding of each.

Dissociation is a hard concept and phenomenon to pin down. This is partly because, unlike repression, it effects a number of different functions of the mind, the effects being present in different combinations and strengths. For instance, dissociation often effects level of consciousness. And yet a pure change in level of consciousness, for instance as one gets sleepy, does not seem like a good example of dissociation. And mental contents are kept from consciousness and apart from each other also in repression and in denial and in other situations such as conscious suppression, not the mention the splitting seen in borderline disorders. So we could ask, how do these situations differ from what happens in dissociation? As a tentative definition, I would propose that dissociation involves the partial or total inaction of the ego functions of integration and differentiation, at one or more of the levels at which they operate. This is not particularly original, but it may be worthwhile, and clarify our understanding of dissociation, if we seek to specify what we mean by this conceptualization, and think through some of the implications of this idea.

If we define dissociation as the shutting down of integrative and differentiation processes at various levels of their functioning, several things are clarified. It makes comprehensible why dissociation involves the combination of things being kept separate—because of the lack of normal integrative functions—and the weird feeling, since consciousness loses its normal synthesis and unity. It also explains the changes to various aspects of conscious experience—caused by the effects of this same disruption in the integrative and differentiation processes on such functions as memory and perception. And it explains why only some problems with these functions feel like dissociation: it is only those problems related to changes in integration and differentiation that feel this way. If one loses an aspect of memory or perception, let's say through brain injury or dementia, we would not call this dissociation. Even if one suffered a purely functional loss, for instance of memory in repression or a fugue or amnesic state, or of vision in hysterical blindness, it does not have the character of dissociation. A loss of perception or memory may be alarming but doesn't have the specific strangeness, as well as the sense of disconnection, that we associate with dissociation. Because integration and differentiation are so central to so many other functions, their partial loss has wide ranging effects, and often feels strange or weird. But it is only when difficulties in other functions are a product of the disablement of integration and differentiation that we think of dissociation.

We should distinguish this disablement also from the splitting that we see especially in borderline disorders. Here our previous comparisons of the primary, secondary, and zero process modes of mental functioning come to our aid. As I will describe in the next chapter, borderline splitting ensues with a weakening of primal repressions and the invasion of the ego by the mode of functioning of the primary process. There is a lack of synthesis in the primary process between different emotional trends such as love and hate, while the lack of integration in the zero process is between various aspects of an experience, such as Joyce's between the feel of the grass on her back and her fear and other parts of her rape, and between her rape and the rest of her life. Borderline splitting does not have effects on level of consciousness or other ego functions in the same manner as dissociation, because in dissociation an ego function central to so many other functions is put out of commission, while in borderline splitting, a functioning ego is invaded to a variable extent by a different mode of functioning, related to a lack of synthesis between emotional trends. (These brief comments don't do justice to the complexity of the relations between these two quite different processes. The discussion of borderline splitting in the next chapter will hopefully help clarify things.)

Another source of confusion with respect to dissociation is that in many instances, the deficits in integration anddifferentiation of dissociation are combined with these other defenses, often in complex structures. An example would be Cordelia's combination of repression and dissociation of the feelings and memories from the many months after her mother had died. One could of course refer to all of these combinations defenses as dissociation, but I don't see anything to be gained by this, and a good deal of clarity to be potentially lost. Using the narrower definition of dissociation allows us to better understand its relation to other processes. This definition also allows us to understand why trauma leads to dissociation, since the general shutting down of higher-level ego processes during trauma effects the integrative and differentiation processes especially severely.

At the same time, we can see that the traumatic process is not just one big dissociation. In relation to this I would like to correct a conceptualization that I had suggested in my book on defenses. There I (2009, pp. 141–145) had defined primary dissociation, following a suggestion by Van Der Kolk et al. (1996), as a passively suffered process, taking place during trauma, in which the shutdown of various ego functions took place leading to the formation of zero process memories. I now feel that this is too broad, because the shutting down of such functions as sublimation of drives, verbal abilities, or the ability to abstract, during trauma cannot be part of dissociation. I say this because there are other examples of dissociation, for instance in hypnosis or the use of secondary dissociation as a defense, where these deficits are not present, and yet we recognize them right away as examples of dissociation. I think there is a primary dissociation in trauma, but it involves only the shutting down of the integrative and differentiating functions, not other aspects of the traumatic breakdown. I use the descriptor "primary" in order to differentiate the passively suffered breakdown of these functions during the shattering effects of trauma, from the more active deactivation of them for various purposes, defensive and adaptive. These latter active dissociations, which are most easily referred to simply as dissociation, are an important part of our normal everyday functioning. Primary dissociation, on the other hand, is a more extreme and less common phenomenon. Later dissociations can be conditioned by, and modelled on, it. Or they can stand alone, as one form of adaptive regression.

In order that we can have a more concrete idea of what all this refers to, let's look at an example. I described previously how Peggy felt that she was living not just in the present, but also in the scary and weird world of her psychotic mother. This has the feel of dissociation. We can get a sense of the nature of the defense by the nature of the resistance we met in analyzing it. When I talked about this other world that she lived in, Peggy at times would join in a discussion of it, but then would make a face, of distress and disgust, and move on to other topics. There did not seem to be a strong force keeping the two realities apart, as Peggy could with not too much trouble access the second reality. There seemed rather to be a combination of avoidance and of an original separation of this set of feelings and memories from her present day experience. I would infer that the original separation was a product of primary dissociations related to Peggy's traumas.

Peggy's later traumatization at the hands of her psychopathic husband was also very consequential in its effects on her but this other world, this other her that was dirty and unloved and so different from everyone else, had been with Peggy since her childhood. She tried not to pay attention to it, and did not explicitly link it with childhood incidents and interactions with her mother. The interesting thing about this was that when we talked of some of the awful feelings from the times with her mother, she would then make the link to the feeling of being different from everyone in the present, and when I pointed out more explicitly that she seemed to live in these two worlds she said "it's always been like that. I've always felt on the outside." When I suggested that the feeling of being on the outside and unable to join with the others might carry forward the feeling she had as a child with her mother, Peggy said it felt the same.

Of course, the evidence for the origin of Peggy's dissociation in the primary dissociation of her original traumas comes not from one interchange but from many, as well as from the whole course of her therapy, in which the non-integration of this dirty, unloved Peggy decreased as we constructed some of her early traumas. I described the particular interchanges, however, as examples that offer a glimpse of the nature of dissociation. Peggy herself brought out the existence of this other set of feelings and when I followed up, or when I brought it up, she might make a face at being reminded of it, but the insights did not seem new to her. Even as some more specific connections might come up, they did not seem to surprise her, but she rather reacted as if hearing something she already knew. What did seem new to her was connecting these different worlds, or the different elements in each world. The memories connected to the present day feelings were not so much blocked from consciousness, as not connected in Peggy's mind with other sets of memories, self images, and experiences.

The basic disconnection that is at the heart of primary dissociation is often obscured by various mental actions performed in order to help maintain the disconnection. In the above example avoidance, one of the most common of these, was especially in evidence. There are many others. For example splitting of the ego, at least in the form described by Freud (1940), involves a powerful denial combined with the dissociative lack of integration. And the separation of different alters (identities) in dissociative identity disorder (DID) involves the use of a powerful counterforce, the zero process version of repression, compounded with dissociation, to produce the separation and the amnestic barriers between alters. But I am getting ahead of myself here. The tale of the different forms of splitting—those that use primary dissociation and those that don't—is a long and complex one. Splitting of the identity will be conceptualized and illustrated in the last section of this chapter, and splitting in borderline disorders will be detailed in chapter four. We have to start at the beginning of this tale, in which there are different functions and aspects of the mind connected together at many levels, and also kept apart at many levels. This dance happens functionally at each moment of our lives, and also developmentally as the range and depth of these processes of integration and differentiation generally grows, even into middle age when many other functions, such as various forms of memory, decline.

In trauma these crucial functions are put out of commission to a great extent and, as a product of this, in the wake of trauma an area of reduced integration/differentiation, which I have called the zero process, comes into existence. These islands of zero process functioning exhibit primary dissociation within the island, in that their bits and pieces of content are not properly connected or differentiated. This primary disconnection is also present in relation to elements outside of the island. This was what Peggy was exhibiting when she described this other reality she always lived with.

In relation to her traumas Peggy displayed not only dissociation but many other defenses, of which I have described repression in some detail. In trauma there is always also a use of secondary dissociation that is built on the primary dissociation of the trauma. Secondary dissociation is an active process, which is modelled on the passively suffered primary form. People who experience ongoing trauma learn how to use this mechanism early on. Peggy pictured herself at the foot of the bed, looking at what was going on when her mother sexually abused her. At other times she would simply be somewhere else in her mind as this happened. We can of course look at things from different perspectives or daydream while something else is going on in the normal course of things, but Peggy took it one step further, as she partially and temporarily and actively shut down the normal integration to a greater extent than would be normal, so that she could more fully escape being present in the experience. This trauma-derived active dissociation can come to dominate the traumatized person's life. It is always there to some extent, and often will be combined with other defenses to form compounds.

It is worthwhile distinguishing the working of various different defenses that deal with different aspects of the same material, such as a set of traumas subject to both repression and dissociation and avoidance, from defenses in which different processes or methods of psychic action are more tightly bound one to the other. I proposed in my book on defenses (2009) to call these latter **compound defenses**. As always, we infer the inner nature or mechanism of a defense by the sorts of resistances and reactions we encounter when we try and get to what lies behind the defense. In the case of Peggy's avoidance and dissociation we can see them working in concert, to defend the same split-off zero process memories of the traumas, but we could analyze the defenses separately, as we could Peggy's repression of her trauma of sexual abuse and the other denials and dissociations of the incidents. In the case of compound defenses one finds it impossible to analyze the different mechanisms separately, from which one infers that they are tightly bound together, although why this is so is not clear. It is perhaps related to something of their history. The two main classes of compound defenses that I have been able to discern are those which combine various psychic actions, such as repression or denial, with dissociation, and the large class of obsessional defenses, which combine a drive derived counterforce similar to repression with various ego functions or activities. (As an example the defense of isolation combines the differentiating function with this counterforce.)

By defining dissociation as involving the disabling of the integrative/differentiating functions, we can also understand both why it has come to be so closely connected with trauma, and at the same time why it does not need trauma as a causative factor. We after all use regression in the form of a partial shutting down of various functions as part of our normal everyday life. Going to sleep involves the most thoroughgoing of regressions, and yet we have to be able to manage this at least once a day, while everything from having sex to enjoying a movie involves a partial shutting down of at least some regular functions such as reality testing and the differentiation between fantasy and reality. Do these involve dissociation? It depends on how wide we want to cast the net of our definition. Because the mental actions that are more obviously dissociations, such as Peggy's during her sexual abuse, also involve the shutting down of certain functions, and distortions in our contact with reality, we may be tempted to cast our net widely and include in the definition of dissociation other instances of this shutting down and distortion of contact with reality. I think this only leads to confusion. Better to define dissociation as the partial shutting down of the integration/differentiation functions, and note that very often this is combined with other regressions and temporary suspensions of other ego functions.

Another phenomenon which involves dissociation is hypnosis. But here too, there are other things going on. Freud (1921) described the putting of the hypnotist in the place of the person's ego ideal, with the hypnotized subject putting themselves in the position of the child who is guided by and in awe of the idealized parent/hypnotist. Gill and Brenman (1961) describe a basic characteristic of hypnosis as involving a regression in the service of the ego, a group of phenomena described by Ernst Kris (1950) in which regression is used for adaptive purposes, and ego control and direction are maintained. Kris was originally an art historian, and he first formulated this important concept in relation to understanding the process of artistic creativity. It has very wide application. Psychoanalysis and psychoanalytic psychotherapy use this process—in fact depend on it—and those who have trouble with it either because they cannot allow the regression (obsessional characters) or because they cannot control it (borderline and psychotic patients) have trouble with analysis.

Gill and Brenman described two phases of hypnosis in relation to controlled regression. The first phase of induction, and the second of hypnosis proper. In the induction phase the hypnotist performs certain actions that destabilize the subject's usual functioning. For instance, they may suggest that the subject's arm will rise without them willing it. In fact all of our physical movements are put into action prior to any conscious decision to perform the action. But as the subject notices that this is the case, their sense of the unity of their conscious will and the movements of their body, an illusory but strongly held belief, is broken, and their sense of reality and of their identity is disrupted. It is at this point that the hypnotist offers themselves as the strong parental figure, and the regression is organized in this way, with the hypnotist taking over certain control and narcissistic functions that normally rest with the superego, heir to the ideal, perfect, perfectly strong, and narcissistically invested parent of early childhood. This dynamic and structural situation is quite common and plays a crucial part in interpersonal and group psychology—for instance it underlies the lasting hold abusers have on the abused, and that authoritarian leaders have on their followers. The point I want to make by touching on these dynamics is that dissociation is only part of a set of dynamics and of structural shifts that take place in hypnosis.

While in these more complex processes dissociation is only one part of the picture, it plays a starring role in attempts to manage trauma while it is happening and in keeping at bay memories of it after the fact. The maneuvers that Peggy performed, where she was looking at herself from a distance as the abuse took place, or that Joyce performed of going completely somewhere else in her mind as the rape became more and more violent, are known to anyone who works with abuse victims. In these maneuvers the person learns from the trauma and the zero process. When traumas first take place, the person suffers passively from primary dissociation, as their integrative and differentiating functions shut down. After this most people take things into their own hands and try to stay one step ahead of the trauma, and their abuser, by shutting down these functions as part of an effort to keep from being as effected by the trauma and to keep the trauma from effecting the rest of their lives. Peggy separated out not just the sexual abuse, but her mother's crazy behaviour, and the lack of real warmth and connection, from the rest of her life through this dissociation, in which she interfered with the integrative and differentiation processes that would otherwise have connected them with her life beyond her mother. Peggy lived her life outdoors, going on adventures in the countryside, playing with her sister and friends, and not thinking at all of what awaited her back home. This dissociation continued throughout her life, as she described living in two worlds, and also demonstrated it by her reactions in the therapy.

There are two points I would like to make about Peggy's dissociation. First, unlike the passively suffered primary dissociation of trauma, Peggy clearly gave up only some of her integrative functions and organizing functions. In order to shut down the integration and connections and differentiations between her traumas and the rest of her life, there had to be some kind of higher-level organization of these maneuvers. In this important way, in the maintenance of some ego control, Peggy's use of dissociation differed from the primary dissociation visited on her by her traumas. On the other hand, and the second point I would like to make about this dissociation, is that while it was under ego control, the control only went so far, and the dissociation was rigidly maintained. The control did not extend to being able to give up the dissociation based on changing circumstances. Even when she did not need the dissociation, even when she was a capable adult who could have dealt with what was dissociated, no choice was possible. This is of course the nature of defenses: they either were at the start, or later become, automatized, and are also protected from conscious awareness by defenses. This may seem like an obvious point to an analyst or dynamic psychotherapist but it is worth emphasizing nonetheless, in order to distinguish dissociation used as a defense, from the very common situations, such as enjoying a movie or enjoying sex, in which the controlled relaxation of integration and/or differentiation is under much more flexible and extensive ego control. This control is still unconscious in the descriptive sense, but there is no strong defense at work, and so the dissociation can be flexibly given up or used again as needed, depending on circumstances. Almost by definition, true defenses cannot flexibly accommodate to circumstances—which is why they cause so many problems.

For instance, the example of driving somewhere quite automatically, thinking of other things while you are doing it, and at the end of the drive not remembering how you got there, is often presented as an everyday example of dissociation. However, it differs from Peggy's defensive use of dissociation in that in driving while thinking of other things, the keeping separate of the two activities and perceptions is quite flexibly reversible based on current circumstances. If it started to rain heavily and one needed to pay attention because of the dangerous driving conditions, or if there was a detour because of construction, one would not continue in one's thinking of other things and crash the car or drive right into the part of the road under construction. One would "wake up" to the situation and pay more conscious attention to it as needed. In the situation of driving without conscious awareness, the higher-level organizing functions are generally operative, and controlling when the person allows the driving to happen automatically and when conscious attention is called into action.

In these brief remarks on dissociation I have not covered the large literature on the topic. My aim has not been to present an exhaustive coverage of all aspects of dissociation, but rather to highlight the ways in which it relates to the characteristics of the zero process. To summarize: I have proposed the term primary dissociation for the loss of integrative and differentiating functions that occurs as part of the traumatic process, and secondary dissociation, or simply "dissociation," for the active shutting down of these functions for defensive purposes. This active defense can be built on the basis of repeating a primary dissociation, in order to manage a trauma, or can be brought about in its own right without traumatic antecedents. Dissociation is often combined with other mechanisms to form compound defenses, some of which will be discussed later. These include splitting of the ego (dissociation plus denial), splitting of the identity (dissociation plus repression-like counterforce), compartmentalization (dissociation plus suppression), and hypnosis-like states of emotional enthrallment and enslavement (dissociation plus narcissistic and superego changes).

Post-traumatic secondary dissociation shown by patients such as Peggy is an example of a type of defense I have designated as a zero process defense. In these, the ego takes over characteristics of the zero process and aspects of the traumatic process that leads to the zero process and uses them for its own purposes. Another example of this is when the person goes numb and shuts down their feeling after the trauma, re-playing the shut down that occurred during the trauma, but keeping this going actively, for years afterwards. Another set of defenses uses one of the main characteristics of the zero process: the fact that its contents, never having been processed into a normal present moment, are not part of the psychical past. The contents of the zero process are always about to happen or just happening, but never fully happen. We turn now to the forms of defense that use this characteristic of post-traumatic memory.

Zero Process Denial and Temporal Shifting

Joyce, whose rape by a colleague was only the beginning of a horrendous ordeal that I will describe in the next section, said, after much analysis of these traumas, that "we have gone over this in so many ways, and I'm convinced that these things happened. And yet I can't believe that they did. They still don't seem real to me." Statements like this are commonly encountered in the therapy of trauma. They often express a denial of the terrible things that have happened, as a way of keeping their full horror at bay. But at this point with Joyce, we had worked through repressions, dissociations, and denials to some extent, and during the sessions where this denial came up, she was not intellectualizing or shifting attention. She knew that the incidents had happened, and seemed yet to also know that they hadn't. She seemed unable to square these two pieces of knowledge. It is tempting to see dissociation and splitting of the ego at work here, in the lack of integration of these two realities. But where did the other reality, that the traumatic incidents had not happened, come from? From Joyce's fantasy life and wishes? But why in this sort of denial is there a different level of certainty than in others where the person has a fantasy that something has not happened?

Having formulated the concept of the zero process it struck me that this attitude of the traumatized made a lot of sense. Joyce said that she felt that the trauma had not happen because it had not. Zero process experiences are unprocessed and thus, in the sense that we usually mean when we say something has happened, the core of the trauma still lived in the future. Of course there was more to Joyce's statement than a description of this zero process reality. It was being used for defensive purposes. However, it was especially experiences where these other defensive aspects had been partially analyzed and neutralized that suggested to me that we have here a basic characteristic of the zero process: its not-yet-happened nature. Interpretation of this aspect of the defense often has the effect of loosening up a denial which has resisted other interpretations, leading to changes in symptoms and behaviour.

It is these changes especially that are convincing in terms of the inference that these denials of trauma use the "not yet happened" nature of the zero process. In Joyce's case I said, "maybe you still don't believe it happened because it hasn't. Maybe its not happening feels so real because it is a true perception of a reality. You haven't yet processed and made real the incidents we are talking about, because they were too horrible and overwhelming." This led to more memories of her captivity coming up in that session and following ones. A number of her memories from the rape—which I described at the beginning of chapter two—turned out to be screens for more deeply repressed ones from her captivity after the rape. As an example Joyce had a memory of white and brown and realized it was the ceiling of the place where she had been held captive, tied up and on her back. She then thought of the memory from the rape of being on her back looking at the sky and clouds, and realized that this both contained and screened the memory from her captivity. The sky expressed a wish for escape from the room. The interpretation of Joyce's zero process denial seemed to facilitate the loosening of her repression of these memories.

As we get into a specific clinical example things always get more complex, as there are many things going on—in this case, one of these things was repression and splitting of identity, which I will detail in the next section. To isolate for now the denial aspect: I have found that it is only by directly giving the zero process reality that the traumatic incidents have not yet happened its full due, that these denials can be analyzed. A more regular interpretation or discussion of the denial might center on how hard it is to accept the reality of what happened, such as the cruelty and sadism of Joyce's captors, and the feelings of abandonment. The interpretation of the nature of the zero process, by noting that the events have not happened yet, adds to these more standard interpretations and empathic responses, by directly bringing to light the nature of the zero process and addressing it as a reality, rather than trying to analyze or interpret it away. Interpreting it away would involve reducing the not-yet-happened nature, by seeing it as a product of a fantasy or wish that the events would not have happened. These motivations certainly make use of the nature of the zero process, but they do not create it—the traumatic process does. I believe that this is why addressing this reality as a given that the person has to deal with, as they have to deal with an external reality which they also did not create, can have such a powerful therapeutic effect. In a sense it involves a deeper empathy, with the zero process nature of the second reality that the person has had to live with for so long. I have heard from a few others who, influenced by my work, have tried these sorts of interventions in addressing traumatic denial, that they have had similar positive results. Therapies that had been stuck, going over the same traumatic events with no movement forward either within or outside of the therapy, began moving on both fronts.

Related to zero process denial is a defense that I have designated as temporal shifting. This defense also makes use of the not-yet-happened nature of the zero process. Zero process memories live in the future, as things that are about to happen. In temporal shifting they are kept in the future and the person lives at a point just before the trauma happened. In this way the full force of the trauma is kept at bay. In fact, the hopelessness and helplessness experienced at the height of the trauma is felt to be avoidable: perhaps this event that lives in the future will happen differently than expected and all will be well. In his paper on fear of breakdown Winnicott (1974) describes a similar situation, in which the breakdown that the person fears in the future has already happened in the material sense, but has not happened psychically. (Scarfone (2006) presents a valuable updated theoretical analysis of Winnicott's idea and of the concept of time and temporality more generally.) Winnicott's view of this process is narrower than mine, as he links it to states of breakdown in infancy that have not been registered psychically. This is a common narrowing of focus, in which the primitive functioning related to trauma is interpreted as evidence for origins in early infancy. The particular patients that Winnicott had in mind may very well have had an early unregistered agony, but seen in a broader context this well known and influential paper is part of a trend within psychoanalysis, in which various aspects of trauma are traced to early infancy and mother-child interactions. I would argue that temporal shifting of the breakdown is present as a characteristic of trauma from infancy to old age. I would also argue that the shift is not based on a non-registration of the event but on a different type of registration, which is certainly deficient in certain qualities of regular registration but that, as I tried to argue earlier in our trip down memory lane in the previous chapter, has aspects of perceptual memory as well as of the other forms of memory.

Temporal shifting is at first not an active defensive activity but a product of the traumatic process and a characteristic of the zero process. The defense of zero process denial uses this shift to the future by taking hold of the psychical fact that the trauma has not yet happened. The defensive use of temporal shifting is ubiquitous in post-traumatic states. The stopping of time, and its shifting, is an important aspect of many conceptualizations of trauma. Among psychoanalysts the French and French Canadians especially have explored the idea of temporality and trauma (eg. Scarfone 2006, 2014, 2015), but many others have fashioned concepts to address this aspect of post-traumatic functioning—for instance Kestenberg (1980, 1993) talks of transposition of the past and the present, and of a time tunnelling that connects the two realms. What the theory of the zero process gives us is a deeper way of connecting specific aspects of the traumatic process and post-traumatic functioning with these temporal peculiarities of trauma, a broader understanding of what this time transposition really means, what its deeper dynamics are, and how best to analyze it.

Cordelia was afraid that she would die or was dying, usually of an ailment related to her belly or stomach. When people she knew or who were close to her developed physical symptoms she jumped to help, quite quickly becoming scared that they were in peril and that she had to save them. She and these others were her ill mother, but in all of these reactions her mother's death, and Cordelia's feelings of despair and de-animation after losing her mother, lay in the future. This is the structure of many traumatic repetitions: the core of the overwhelming is pushed into the future, and the person lives at the point just before all ability to cope and all hope was lost, at a point where things could still turn out differently. Repetition is such a prominent part of the post-traumatic state, that it can blind us to the fact that what looks like a simple repetition is rarely such, but involves a complex dynamic, one part of which involves repeating not the trauma, but the point before it truly overwhelmed the person. In most cases what looks like a repetition is a zero process drive/defense compromise. As well, a common way of dealing with trauma, by sexualizing it, to turn the awful into the exciting, also usually works not on the core of the trauma but on things that immediately precede it, so that sexualization works in tandem with temporal shifting.

How do we know, beyond observation and speculation, that these post-traumatic structures are a product of a specific defense or set of defenses against the drive to re-experience the trauma? One simple but powerful piece of evidence is that direct interpretation of the zero process nature of the defense will start things moving, and lead to more material emerging. I gave an example of this sort of direct interpretation of zero process denial when I said to Joyce that she was right to say that her trauma felt like it had not happened, because it had not. This is a direct interpretation of temporal shifting made use of for the purposes of denial. But in the true temporal shifting defense, one not only denies that the trauma has happened but lives at the point just before the overwhelming, fearing the trauma in the future. Zero process denial and temporal shifting work in concert. The first denies that the event happened in the past, the second pushes it into, or rather keeps it in, the future. An interpretation to Cordelia of the second might be, "what you're afraid will happen to yourself or the people you rush to help is what happened to your mother." This interprets the content, but not the zero process structure. It isn't the exact words that matter, but rather the knowledge and attitude of the therapist. One should not treat the trauma being in the future as only a fantasy or wish, nor just a process of learning that what happened previouslywill happen again. Post-traumatic phobias are often understood in this cognitive, learning sense. In contrast to this, one has to take cognizance of the fact that the trauma being in the future is a psychic reality in a deep structural sense—the traumatic occurrences live in the person's perceptual systems as a second reality.

Thus to Cordelia I said, "your mother's death hasn't yet happened to you. It remains in your future and you keep it there to keep open the possibility that it will all turn out differently." These sorts of interventions led to further material about what Cordelia felt when the repetitions took place, and to further memories of their sources in the past. I also said, "the loss of your mother has crowded out many more realistic possibilities in your future, as it has come to live there, and the time just before that loss has come to dominate your present." The power of these sorts of general interventions to mobilize memories and feelings from both the present repetitions, the past traumas, and their connections, is one piece of evidence for the importance of these temporal shifting defenses in post-traumatic repetitions. The interventions were only part our work on Cordelia's trauma. They served the specific purpose of opening up access to unconscious material, which is what you would expect from any successful defense interpretation. Usually the defense is not just used against the trauma, but for other purposes. In Cordelia's case, it helped postpone the full mourning process. She could and did feel sadness and pain, as we talked of her memories of her mother and of her hearing of her death. But she avoided the release phase of mourning, where there is a de-investment in the lost person and a freeing up of energies. There was always the possibility that her mother would not be permanently lost, because this loss was in the future.

In relation to Cordelia's therapy I described above, in the section on repression, how it was interpretation of her temporal shift defenses that opened up access to the time after she had heard about her mother's death, when she was overwhelmed by feelings of desolation and de-animation. This is a good demonstration of how the interpretation of this defense is not the end of work on the trauma, but often the beginning of explorations of new areas. In the section on repression I went into some detail about our analysis of this repressed and previously unremembered time in Cordelia's life. This led to immediate improvement, with Cordelia feeling less anxious about people's health concerns, and herself having more of an appetite and gaining weight. But within weeks, she started to have mounting anxieties, as well as resistances around coming to appointments and scheduling appointments. In relation to her talking about these mounting anxieties about other people's health, especially one person close to her, I made further comments related to temporality. I said that at the emotional level her mother's death and its aftermath had lived for her especially in the future. This was a repetition of what I had said earlier. But I wondered if, at this point, as this trauma she had kept in her future began to emerge from repression, she was redoubling her efforts to push it into her future, as she became obsessively preoccupied with the health of those around her. She said that she had been feeling "deadful" for the last couple of days. She had meant to say "dreadful." She was having anxiety about losing all of her friends, or that she had already lost them. She was feeling an adrenaline rush, as she worked to save everyone, but this left her feeling in the end exhausted. She then felt shame, for not being able to regulate herself, a feeling that she for the first time linked to the time after her mother's death.

Cordelia came to the next session saying she had felt better immediately after our session. She had been thinking as she came to my office of the mother and daughter who had been in the news who had perished together in a fire. I wondered about her being pulled into her mother's dead state. She thought of her slip of saying "deadful." "I think I was deadful for a year after my mother's death, before I pulled out of it." Her thoughts went to a time in her early twenties, when she developed health problems that were incorrectly diagnosed. She was very despondent then, feeling her life was over just as it was getting started. She was depressed and despondent for a number of months, but then pulled herself up and decided that she would just live with her condition and started travelling. Things improved quickly for her after that. This seemed a reprise of what she had gone through after her mother's death, she realized. She had not gone over this time in her twenties in such detail previously (I'm leaving out the details for reasons of confidentiality), and a lot fell into place when she did so.

In the next session Cordelia said that she felt she was getting on top of the overwhelming feelings. She recounted a dream, in which she was desperate to get to her grandmother. She got into a car in order to get to her, along with her stepmother. Her cellphone flew out of the car, and went backwards. It was a surreal event in the dream. It was as if time itself was flying backwards. Cordelia thought of how she had been so excited as a child to hear that her stepmother was coming to take care of her. This was what snapped her out of her year of despair following her mother's death. But she had been sorely disappointed by her harshness. This she contrasted with her grandmother's warmth and love. She then thought of going in for her appendix operation in later childhood and being certain—not just afraid but certain—that she would die. She has not been eating, she says. She has no appetite. As she talks of eating she thinks of not having enough time to eat. "That is what it feels like. Like I just don't have enough time. Like I don't have enough time to get to my grandmother in the dream. Time is running out." In saying this, Cordelia was pointing to one of the key issues in all trauma: things happen too quickly, before you are ready, and before you can prepare. She thinks of eating, she says. I wonder if it was like taking in her mother, eating her mother. She thinks of her mother taking care of the kids, feeding them.

Two sessions later, Cordelia comes in and almost immediately recounts a dream. "It's related to my mother, I'm sure. It's about my first husband, D. He was ill and hospitalized. He was the age he was when we first met. His present wife was there. I had broken up with him, and he had been ill. I felt a longing to get back together. I had decided to reunite with him, but his wife was in the way. When I went to hold his hand, it was a woman's hand, dry and cracked. I felt guilt that my leaving him had made him get ill." Cordelia first says that she had always thought of D as maternal. This leads her to think of her mother losing weight. She wonders if she felt guilty for going on with her life, as her mother died. This dream is rich in the things that Cordelia was struggling with around her mother and her trauma. There are the clear Oedipal themes, with the woman in the way. But in her associations this was wound around the trauma in different ways. In the previous dream her stepmother seemed somehow to be getting in the way of her getting to her grandmother. The dream of not being able to get to her grandmother was a recurring one, since Cordelia's early twenties. Recurring dreams such as this always contain a replaying of some aspects of a trauma. We knew this in the general sense, but Cordelia's associations to the dream of the husband with the woman's hand led us to specific connections.

Cordelia remembers a sense of shock on seeing her mother in hospital. At first she isn't sure of the veracity of the memories as they come up. She has always had a screen memory of lying with her mother on her hospital bed, facing away from her. Now she remembers how shocked she was to see her mother so gaunt. She had previously been physically robust and full of life. Now she was skin and bones. Cordelia knew her father had not taken the children to see their mother, so as not to upset them. So the change was striking and shocking. The scene was emotional: the last time this young mother would see her young children. And she knew it. What did Cordelia know? She knew her mother's hand was her husband's hand in the dream, gaunt and dry and cracked. She knew something was terribly wrong. We now understand the dreams of trying to get to her grandmother. She felt she should have visited her mother more. She felt she had been kept from visiting her. She felt her mother wasted away because she did not visit. When someone told her that they had this or that symptom her jumping up, anxiously insisting on a remedy, was a replay of the hospital visit and her response to seeing her mother. She was unconsciously transported back there, before the death, shocked and trying to reverse her sense of helplessness. And she was also her mother, losing weight and with no appetite. Cordelia's anorexia had many determinants, but a powerful one was again a time shift: she was her mother, losing weight and gaunt, but still saveable. The details of the last visit with her mother were clung to and replayed. In the session after these memories emerged, Cordelia comes in and says that she had woken up in great anxiety. She had felt that she was just a wisp of a person, who could be blown away by the wind. Her identification with her mother is strengthening. She also says she is avoiding contacting all sorts of people, including people who are ill, whom she would normally visit. The period near the end of her mother's life is starting to repeat, with great force.

I have in these brief sketches of a few sessions tried to give a flavour of how temporal shift defenses fit into the flow of Cordelia's therapy. I have concentrated on the replay of the time before the full hopelessness of the loss of her mother descended upon her. Cordelia unconsciously kept replaying that time, terrible as it was, because there was still hope. Things were bad, but the final die had not been cast. There were also many other dynamics taking place, which therapists familiar with trauma will notice. For instance there was the attempt to turn passive into active, as Cordelia did not visit people rather than not being taken to visit her mother. This also played out as a transference resistance, in trying to cancel sessions and get a break from therapy. And there was the use of guilt as a defense, as she felt she had caused her mother's death by not visiting and not acting to save her. This expressed an unconscious psychic truth, as Cordelia had harboured angry feelings and nasty fantasies about her mother. But these were also brought into the service of denying helplessness: if she was guilty, then she had control of the situation, and could have made things happen differently. All these defenses were made more powerful through temporal shifting. Through the magic of zero process time shifting, the loss had not yet occurred, and the project of changing the past could be transmuted into the much more feasible project of changing the future.

One further type of defense related to temporal shifting that I have written about previously in a more general context (Fernando, 2011) are what I have called **contrast defenses**. I have found a knowledge of these defenses helpful clinically. In a contrast defense, the person avoids things that are too great a contrast with the trauma or other environmental problem, such as deprivation, which has been problematic for them. As an example, a person who has suffered emotional deprivation will avoid, or at least limit their exposure to, loving interactions or, as a compromise, they will allow themselves to receive some love and attention, but say to themselves that after all, the person is only doing this because they feel sorry for them. If they do not do this, if they fully let in the love and caring, they then are overcome by the sadness and pain of their past deprivation. Experiencing the contrast means the bad times are over, and it is time to process them. This avoidance of the contrast is often con-ceptualized in simpler terms, as a pull to repeat what the person has experienced. However, there are usually complex dynamics going on, and an understanding of these touches on what I have been talking about in relation to temporal shifting: that what looks like repetition of a trauma is in reality a more complicated balance in which some forms of repetition are used to defend against worse ones. In the case of temporal shifting, this involves repeating what happened just before the height of the trauma, while in the case of contrast defenses it involves avoiding the opposite to what happened. They both meet at the point of avoiding reliving the trauma, and work together to produce what looks like a simple repetition but is actually a more complex structure.

As an example, Cordelia left a number of relationships when she had been in them for about four years, which looks like a straight repetition of what had happened with her mother's death when she was four. However, in terms of temporal shifting, it became clear that she turned passive into active by leaving them before they left her, and that her leaving at that point left the definitive death of the loved one in the future. She would try to get back together with these men, and she would then find another relationship, all the while keeping the truly overwhelming trauma of definitive loss and emotional breakdown in the future. But why not just stay with these men past four years, to prove to herself that she was safe from loss? Here we run up against the meeting place of temporal shifting and contrast defenses: Cordelia was never safe from the loss of her mother, because it had not happened yet, and was always threatening to happen definitively. If she stayed, having a relationship that, in contrast to the one with her mother, lasted for five or six or more years, then the loss would no longer be in her future—she could not fear that it would happen as it did with her mother, so quickly after their relationship started. There would be nowhere to put the memories of the trauma, and she would start to live them out as a present experience.

Taking the not-yet-happened nature of post-traumatic memories as a reality, as I suggested one do in interpreting zero process denial and temporal shifting, is reminiscent of the work by various psychiatrists and psychologists beginning in the 1970s on the therapy of what was then called multiple personality disorder and is now referred to as dissociative identity disorder (DID). I will mention their names and go into further detail in the next section, but here I would just like to point out that they, often working through trial and error and inventing techniques as they went along, found that one had to address the alternate personalities as realities, rather than try to talk the patient out of their experiences. And not as realities in the sense of a kind of suspension of disbelief, but much more straightforwardly as simple realities—naming the alters, talking to them separately and together, calling them up, and mapping them and their relationships. To many not familiar with DID, this way of going about things can seem either mystical or misleading. It was discovered empirically, however, that only in this way could the traumas be analyzed and the different alters integrated. Here too, as in temporal shifting, the zero process memories face the person as reality. Kluft (2000) described DID as a multiple reality disorder, which dissolves in empathy. Such a view perfectly captures the importance of addressing the trauma patient's zero process reality, and the powerful therapeutic effect of doing so. I see it as a confirmation of the reality and power of the concept to the zero process that it helps us to comprehend, in a non-mystical and realistic manner, both the various forms of defense that I have just described, and some of these seemingly strange aspects of DID and its treatment, that I am about to describe.

Dissociative Identity Disorder and Splitting of the Identity

Patients who seemed to have multiple selves or personalities played an important part in early psychiatric explorations of psychopathology and in the development of ideas of the mind more generally. However, as the first part of the 20th century unfolded, this disorder was not much discussed, and seen either as very rare or as a fiction based on fantasy and acting. In his comprehensive book on what was then called multiple personality disorder Putnam (1989) describes some of this history. He notes that the phenomenology of the disorder, whatever name it has gone under, whether demonic possession or multiple personality disorder, has remained consistent over many centuries. (I would speculate that it has remained so since the birth of the human species.) Putnam suggests it may have been more common in the Middle Ages because of the higher incidence of extreme trauma during those times. For those not familiar with the disorder, Putnam's book is still the best place to start, as it covers all aspects of DID, from its history to its phenomenology, causation, dynamics, and treatment.

It was only in the 1970s and 1980s that there was a more concerted investigation of DID by many clinicians, and the modern understanding of its origins and dynamics emerged. Even then, these investigators were often looked upon suspiciously by many psychoanalysts and general psychiatrists. In the late 1960s Dr. Wilbur, the psychiatrist and psychoanalyst who treated the patient who became known as Sybil, could not get her work published in mainstream academic journals, and her case only became known through a popular book (Schreiber, 1973). What many people find unbelievable, and others find full of dramatic possibilities, is that there could be more than one personality or person inside a single mind. Not only is this unbelievable, it's also not true. But the truth is almost as strange and, while perhaps not as full of dramatic possibilities for novels and films, provides a fascinating window into post-traumatic mental functioning. The modern understandings of DID is that it is a complex ego adaptation to severe chronic trauma, usually trauma that began very early, before three. The specific defenses of this disorder are used by the child to protect themselves and their development from being completely overwhelmed by the traumas. Then, "under the pressure of a variety of developmental factors, secondary structuring and personification by the child of the traumatically induced dissociated states of consciousness leads to development of multiple "personalities." Once dissociative defenses are in place, they may be used preferentially to handle subsequent traumatic experiences as well as to cope with a variety of other developmental issues." (Loewenstein & Ross, 1992, p. 7).

Older ideas were of a few or two alters, one "good", one "bad". Newer ideas, based on more careful investigation, suggest that many alters, ten or twenty or more, is the more common situation. (The idea of two alters, "good" and "bad", may relate to people with borderline splitting being mistakenly diagnosed as DID.) Lowenstein (1993) notes that alters are often not completely separated from each other, but rather are to variable extents present while another is in control. Overlap, interference, and co-presence are common. Most people with DID are intelligent, warm, complex personalities with good ego abilities in many areas, including good capacities for sublimation (Kluft, 2000; Brenner, 2001, 2004). The primary dissociation that I have described as being part of the traumatic process leads to the original split, present in all who have been traumatized. Peggy felt she lived in two different worlds—the regular one and the traumatic childhood one with her psychotic mother. But in DID this original dissociation is used to build up the different alters. There is almost always either serious and early sexual abuse and/or serious threats to life of the person or witnessing mutilations and murders. Sybil's mother hung her upside down and inserted objects in her vagina, and performed other strange sexual acts when she was very young, as an example. This was only one of many traumas inflicted on her, in the context of a very strange mother who was her main caretaker. Along with the depth of trauma, it seems to be the lack of any reprieve, or of a person who provides psychological care and safety, even for some of the time, that pushes towards the full development of separate alters to deal with the situation.

There are a few things to consider here, and I will take them up one at a time. First I will discuss the basic connection between DID and the zero process. Then I will briefly touch on developmental considerations, which will lead to a deeper look at the causation and dynamics of the barriers between different alters that lead to their independence from each other. In relation to this last, I will present further material from Joyce, the patient whose brutal rape began chapter two. In chapter five, on technique, I will consider the idea that splitting of the identity in less severe form is part of most serious traumas—a fact with important implications for developing more powerful treatment techniques.

First, the basic connection between DID and the zero process: Kluft has often (2000, also in personal communications) talked of DID as a multiple reality disorder. This conception of the disorder is a key point of contact with the theory of the zero process. DID involves the survival into the present, not as memories but as functioning present realities, of feelings, perceptions, and attitudes from the past, organized into entities that behave as if they are separate. These entities display some of the key characteristics of zero process structures, such as introjects, that I have discussed. But these characteristics are taken to an extreme in DID, which is dominated by the zero process. This is not to say that everything about the alters and the dynamics of DID can be reduced to the functioning of the zero process, but it is clear that in this disorder higher-level ego functions use characteristics of the zero process for adaptive purposes. The presence of memories as present realities living at the perceptual end of the mind, which push for expression (the zero process drive) is the problem with which trauma leaves us. Out of this problem these creative and resilient individuals craft a solution: around each of these alternate realities—specific incidents, or a series of similar incidents, or specific feelings or impulses—they build a separate alternate part of themselves. Each alter is built like a pearl around the grains of zero process memories. These give the alter its sense of being a present reality. In fact, not just the sense or fantasy, but the reality of being another present lived experience. The zero process drive for immediate expression of the post-traumatic memories would explain the push for existence and expression, including behavioural expression, of their reality by each alter. Putnam (1989) notes that alters are not ambivalent in their attitudes. They only have one opinion and one attitude, and in this betray that they are not complete personalities but rather are derived from zero process memories, which are simple realities which exist as they always have, as an immediate experience. He also notes that alters have a simple transference, with only one emotional note and attitude—again very different from the complex, layered, and ever-shifting transferences seen with whole people, and again easily explained as derived from the frozen traumatic incidents that are the source of the alter and of the transference.

Many of the seemingly strange and mysterious aspects of DID make sense when viewed through the lens of the zero process and its characteristics. At the same time DID can give us deeper insight into these characteristics, much like many of the features of psychosis and of borderline disorders, which involve the invasion of the ego by deeper emotional layers of the mind, allow us a window into the workings of the primary process. Having said this allows me to propose a crude, but I believe illuminating, differentiation between borderline personality disorder (BPD) and DID: BPD involves the invasion of important parts of a person's functioning by the primary process, while DID involves the invasion of important parts of a person's functioning by the zero process. We can take as an example the splitting seen in BPD versus the dissociated alters of DID. The former demonstrates what Freud discovered about the primary process through his study of dreams and neuroses: that in the primary process emotional trends, such as love and hate, exist happily side by side, without a sense of contradiction or a need to integrate them or find some sort of compromise. In BPD, splitting refers to a view of the world in which people are either all good or all bad, and in which the loved and all good can suddenly turn into the hated and all bad. Experienced therapists know that it is a worrying sign when a patient starts to laud them and their abilities right at the first session, even as they tell them of all the terrible things their horrible therapists from the past have done. This split can and will reverse at some point, usually quite abruptly. It is based upon a lack of integration of love and hate, and a lack of stabilization of more modulated investment in others. This borderline splitting is very different from the split between different alters in DID, which is based not on a lack of emotional integration but upon a lack of integration of different external traumatic experiences, now reflected in unintegrated parts of the person. In BPD a lack of internal integration is projected outwards, as the person reacts to the world as all good or all bad, while in DID an original lack of integration of external experiences is internalized and reflected in internal divisions.

Let's take another capacity—reality testing. Lowenstein (1993) notes that the phenomenology of DID can often mimic psychosis. It can include hallucinations of voices (from the other alters), as well as other classic psychotic experiences of being passively influenced such as thought insertion and withdrawal, influences on the body, and "made" feelings, thoughts, and volitional acts. Psychological testing does not demonstrate a true thought disorder, however, and in fact shows psychologically complex individuals with whole object relations and excellent self observing capacities. It is easy enough to reconcile these contradictions if we realize that all of these psychotic seeming reactions relate to the intrusion of another unprocessed reality into the present reality. This isn't the whole story, as the alters then build themselves based on other experiences, and control the person or talk to them, leading to the voices and passive influence experiences. But the core of the loss of touch with regular present day reality is based on the presence of another reality. The resemblance to psychosis can lead to some diagnostic problems, if more careful assessments are not done. Putnam (1989) and Brenner (2001, 2004) note that the decline in the diagnosis of DID coincided with the new descriptions of schizophrenia, and they wonder whether many of those suffering from DID were simply assessed as schizophrenic and put in back wards of asylums. Brenner describes specific cases where a patient diagnosed as schizophrenic was found to have DID. The reader may remember Niederland's (1965) freezing patient described near the beginning of chapter two, who seemed psychotic.

In the case of BPD, the ability to be aware of and test reality, and the basic functions that serve this ability, are intact, as they are in DID (compared to their impairment in psychosis). But in BPD this intactness, and even at times very good functioning in certain more neutral situations such as in a professional role, does not hold up in closer relationships and situations where emotions are heightened. At these times fantasy and wish are mistaken for reality. This can be very striking and at times make the borderline, for very different reasons than someone with DID, seem psychotic. As an example, a patient may insist that you have been very angry at them, and raised your voice to them in the last session. They can seem so sure that you can start to question your own memory of the events. Of course such a situation could be caused by the reliving of a trauma—only the total situation will tell the difference. But in the case of BPD, this distortion of reality is based on a specific characteristic of the primary process that Freud described already in 1900 in the Interpretation of Dreams. In the primary process, there is no differentiation between wish, fantasy, and reality. Thus in situations in which emotions and the wishes and fantasies driven by them run high, which would be especially situations of close relationship with someone, this aspect of the primary process comes to the fore, and the reality testing of someone with BPD is impaired.

This brings up another interesting difference between DID and BPD: in BPD the various aspects of the disorder, such as the splitting and mistaking of fantasy for reality, increase markedly in close relationships, and are usually at their worst in romantic and sexual relationships. In the case of DID, there is no specific connection. Whatever is connected in concrete ways with the traumas and the alters based on them will exacerbate things. Of course interpersonal interactions are a likely culprit, but so are such things as anniversary reactions, or accidental happenings that trigger memories from the traumas. The reader may wonder about the mixed situation, of a BPD sufferer with significant trauma, maybe even DID? Certainly this cannot be uncommon. It is possible that descriptions of DID involving two alters, one bad and one good, involve this kind of mixture of primary process and zero process dynamics, as do some cases of extremely complex DID with proliferating alters that do not stabilize.

What leads to the specific outcome of DID? And how are the special structural characteristics of DID built up in the mind, and maintained? Let's approach these questions by looking at developmental aspects. There are reports in the literature of DID developing in children (e.g.,—the many contributions in Kluft, 1985a). An instructive case is reported by Riley and Mead (1988), of a child of three who developed a separate personality, in response to being sent back from a stable guardian mother to her biological mother who, along with the boys in a generally very terrifying environment, sexually and psychologically abused her. She had told people about it, but still was sent back by the court to the biological mother. She developed a younger girl alter, Lila, who knew about the abuse and seemed to contain some of the memories. There are videos of the child becoming the two different personalities, with the distracted gaze as she switched, impairments of memory, and other hallmarks of DID. The authors note, as have others (e.g., Kluft, 1985b) that the symptoms were much more easily treated in this child and in children in general, who seem to have a weak investment in the multiplicity as such. In adults the alters have a strong narcissistic investment in their own separate existence. It is well understood that the development of alters has its own history. They usually only become fully separated and invested in their own separateness during adolescence and early adulthood. This is not to say that there are not well formed and independent alters before this—in fact there usually are. But the fact that there is not as much difficulty in integrating the alters with each other and the main personality suggests that something is added to strengthen the separation during and just after adolescence. This something is not far to seek, as we know it as the normal formation of a more strongly held and separate identity and sense of self in adolescence and early adulthood. One of the main mechanisms through which this identity development is accomplished is through the setting up of stronger self/other boundaries using aggression or, to be more precise, partially neutralized aggressive drive energy.

At the beginning of phases when this self/other boundary is being established—in early toddlerhood and early adolescence—the aggression towards caretakers and its connection to establishing independence is quite evident. The two-year-old will stamp their feet and say "no" on principle to whatever is offered or asked, while the 12-year-old will demonstrate their higher sophistication as they now look with disdain upon their parents, who have almost overnight become stupid and ugly and clumsy and a source of unending and unendurable embarrassment. At these times the aggression has a life or death feel, and there is some truth to this, as the life of the person's identity and sense of a separate self is at stake. What is interesting also is the way in which, as time goes on and the child matures out of each of these stages, the aggression against the caretakers decreases and often largely disappears, as the sense of a separate self becomes more secure. At this point, the use of more modulated, neutralized aggression to maintain self/other boundaries is not so obvious, but it is a relatively secure inference from many lines of evidence. Among these are the way that a breakdown in the ability to neutralize aggression, as happens in schizophrenia, leads to a breakdown in the most basic boundaries of the self, so that even its differentiation from inanimate objects can be lost. Other structures in the mind, specifically repressions and reaction formations which keep id impulses and anal wishes to mess at bay, break down at the same time and to the same extent in schizophrenia, leading us to infer a similar derivation of these internal structures and self/other differentiation. In those with secure self/other boundaries, when these boundaries are threatened, as they are for instance in psychological abuse, anger is the immediate response – anger that is quite similar to when a repression is threatened with an interpretation—evidence again of the derivation of these self/other boundaries from partly neutralized aggression. Working more quietly than the aggression, new, deeper and more stable, libidinal investments in the self, much of it coming from powerful investments in the parents that are partially withdrawn, also take place.

We can infer that what is added to the primary and secondary dissociation of trauma in DID, to bring about the clear separation of the alters, is partially neutralized aggression to form self/self boundaries, and libidinal investments in the alter, in much the same manner as self/ other boundaries are formed. One does not need the theory of the zero process to see this, but this theory makes more comprehensible how it can be done. According to this theory what is left after trauma are not memories but experiences. In a radical sense, the material world of the frozen present of the trauma invades the intrapsychic world, but remains at the perceptual end of the mind. This is different from internalization of the world in memories and fantasies and wishes, and different from the use of all of these to build up our internal working models of the world, which do not remain as perceptions but move deeper, into the regular memory and representational systems of the mind. These ideas of zero process theory will lead us, I believe, to see the inner object world and internal objects as hybrid phenomenon, made from a world that lives in the perceptual end of the mind, and one deeper in the memory systems and other parts of the mind.

The zero process itself is a hybrid, but of a different sort—a piece of internal psychic reality, and yet behaving like a piece of external reality and lived immediate experience. Because of this, the structuring of it in DID seems also to be of a hybrid nature: sharing something with both the internal structuring of repression and the external structuring of the demarcation of the self from others and the world. Both of these structuring activities have almost the same mechanism, of using partially neutralized aggression to push something—whether a person or a powerful sexual drive—away, and keep it away or at a distance. In DID this mechanism rides on top of the basic dissociation—the lack of integration—of the contents of the zero process. I would suggest that it is another example of what I have called a compound defense—that is, a defense in which different psychic mechanisms or actions are tightly coupled together. While I present these ideas about splitting of the identity as speculation informed by theory, they were arrived at more directly, through observing the nature of the resistances we meet when trying to analyze the separation of different identities formed during trauma. There are secondary defenses of avoidance and denial that often need to be dealt with first, but then as one gets closer, one meets the characteristic burst of anger heralding the breaching of a counterforce, whether repression or self/other differentiation. But only when the dissociation is analyzed at the same time as this counterforce does the split identity give way. I will expand on these brief comments in chapter five, on trauma therapy, where I will present clinical material related to the analysis of splitting of the identity. Here I will present some preliminary material to give a flavour of splitting of the identity.

This material is not from a classic case of DID. My clinical experience and technical abilities on this score are limited, and what I have seen would not add anything or go as deeply as the experience of others who have presented cases in the literature. Rather this material, from the psychoanalysis of Joyce, whose memories of rape began chapter two, involve events from an adult trauma that demonstrate some dynamics of splitting of the identity. Just to give some background: Joyce had suffered much more than her share of trauma. She had been sexually molested by a friend of the family in early childhood, around the age of 5. It was clear he had touched her, and she had told her mother, who had told her to try to avoid him and not to make a fuss. The memories of what else had happened somehow never became clear through most of Joyce's four to five times weekly psychoanalysis. Had he later trapped her in his car, in the parking lot of an abandoned industrial building, and raped her? Had he taken her to his cabin, and raped her there, in a small dark bedroom? The reason for the blurriness of all this emerged as we uncovered what had happened to Joyce after the adult rape that I described previously. It turned out that many of the memories that seemed to be from the early time had been projected backwards from the time of her adult rape and captivity and abuse afterwards. Little pieces of memory from that later time were located in the earlier one and put together with actual memories from childhood to form a kind of screen for the adult trauma.

Joyce had suffered other traumas in childhood, including sexual abuse by a pedophile neighbour. On the other hand, she had a very loving mother who was also excellent at building up Joyce's independence and ego capacities, giving her warm loving support but also not jumping in too quickly to help her do things, and thus building up her own ego capacities and independence. It is hard to disentangle constitution from early interactions as causative factors, but it was my impression that Joyce had a very high capacity to sublimate and use her basic drives and affects, probably based on her parenting and constitution, which spared her the self attack that often follows trauma, and made her uniquely resilient among the patients I have seen. To give just one example: Joyce would go to bed during times of the sexual abuse by the pedophile neighbour, by picturing herself stabbing him, or more playfully smashing his head as if it were a pumpkin. This gave sufficient outlet for the dammed up aggression and feelings of helplessness for Joyce to go to bed easily. She never felt any guilt about these fantasies that I could detect over many years of intensive analysis, even though through all the years I treated her, I never saw anything but that she had a very finely tuned and well functioning sense of morality, and moral actions that flowed from this.

After a number of years, we had breakthroughs in analyzing Joyce's childhood traumas when we were able to undo certain key repressions. The earlier abuse, which remained so obscure, had become linked to Oedipal fantasies and wishes which were then powerfully repressed. The abuser was a charismatic man who Joyce both admired and hated. The later abuse by the neighbourhood pedophile had led to Joyce developing rage against her beloved mother as she became aware that she knew what was going on. She had repressed both the rage and her knowledge that her mother knew. We also uncovered and analyzed the repression of the time when the abuse had started, before she had stabilized herself and developed her adaptive dissociations and compartmentalizations. During these months she was in terrible shape, completely overwhelmed and not knowing where to turn. It is probably in these sorts of situations that children will start to form alters. But Joyce was somewhat older, entering a stage where there is normally rapid growth of intellectual and defensive functions (by age seven), she was resilient, and she had a loving and supportive mother (except in the area of protecting her from abuse, which most likely related to the mother being repeatedly gang raped by soldiers when young, and helplessly watching them do the same to her sister and mother). So Joyce repressed memories of this early stage and restructured her life and mind to manage what was going on. I won't go into detail about how these repressions were analyzed, except to say that the analysis of the transference played a key part in the work. The work took many years of four to five times weekly analysis.

I very much want to give more details of Joyce's development and childhood abuse, as there is much to learn from them. But considerations of confidentiality and of space limit me, and I will now discuss what happened after her adult rape. I have described how a senior colleague from business had lured her into his garden and raped her violently. For a long time, what happened afterwards was left vague, but it was assumed that she fled. There were things that had happened afterwards which made us both wonder about this simple scenario. I will not describe these details for reasons of confidentiality. It was later, after we had stopped the analysis, that something happened that led Joyce back to me. I have not yet described what brought her to analysis in the first place. Partly, she wanted to work through the sexual abuse traumas that she had kept to herself for so long. She had a sense they had something to do with why she ended up with narcissistic and difficult men, who were abusive physically or psychologically, although not in the extreme manner of her childhood. She also found that in certain situations she simply would lose the ability to stand up for herself, even though she was quite good at doing this under most circumstances. And, she had not pursued the business that she had been so good at, dropping it and any further connections to it after the adult rape. The first two of these things had changed quite a bit with our analysis of Joyce's childhood traumas and repressions, but the third had not. There was a sense that even in terms of her being triggered in situations with narcissists, there was something that was hidden from us. But she was as a practical matter doing very much better, and so we brought the analysis to an end.

Joyce called me when circumstances forced her hand, in terms of doing something in the type of business that she had so completely avoided since the adult rape. This led to intense anxiety and avoidance of what she had to do. She knew it was part of a phobic avoidance we had discussed and had linked to the adult rape, as she had not had the phobia prior to that. In fact many aspects of her life had changed after the rape. This in one sense did not seem so surprising given its brutality. We had also thought that it had reactivated various aspects of her childhood traumas. Joyce's confidence that she could protect herself, which had come from sending her abuser away in childhood by threatening him with exposure, was shattered by what happened to her as an adult. Still, when Joyce came back to therapy, she had a feeling there was more. And I had to agree. The intensity of the anxiety suggested it, as did the various things she had done in the immediate months after the adult rape. And, she noted, it was more and more clear to her that she had been functioning quite well until this attack. Why had it all changed not just so suddenly, but so deeply? It was almost as if she was a different person afterwards. We both knew that this wasn't true, that she had remained essentially who she was. And yet it was true in a way we could not quite catch hold of. We discovered in the resumed therapy that followed that what had been profoundly altered was her relationship with herself.

As we talked about the time of the rape in young adulthood, Joyce had a number of very strong reactions to certain situations. In one it was the taste of some food that triggered overwhelming fear and anxiety. She was afraid, almost to the point of paranoia, of friends who were trying to help her when she went home after eating the food. She had trouble speaking and also had other physical symptoms, which made her friends think she was having a medical emergency. Somehow, through all the fear and confusion, she knew this wasn't the case, and that she was living out something. Over the next few days, she could not lie in bed, but had to immediately get up, driven by a terror she could not fathom. But she knew it had something to do with being restrained. We had wondered if something more had happened after the rape, and she was getting the feeling that she had been held hostage by this man and some others. She did not want to think this could be true. Our approach to this, the uncovering of what had actually happened, and our working through of it, took a few years of therapy. With the reaction described above, what came to her is that she had been drugged. She had been offered something when she first visited the senior colleague's house, which was connected to the food she had eaten that had triggered the intense anxiety episode. "In a way it makes sense. I had always blamed myself for not listening to my gut. I usually listened to it, and I was getting a funny feeling as I was sitting there with him, and he was asking me if people kept in touch, if they would miss me ... and about my parents. But I know now, I was feeling woozy, like I was feeling at the meeting. Everything was confused. I'm not sure if that's true, even though I know it is."

Joyce got confused about appointment times, and vacation dates. This was new for her. She had very easily remembered these sorts of things during the previous analysis. She got confused and dizzy going up the steps from my basement home office after an appointment. Then it happened again coming in. I asked her what came to mind and she associated to memories that she had mentioned long ago of climbing up the steps to her first abusers country house as a very young girl. But she realized she had confused two things. These were steps to somewhere else. Was it where she had been taken after the rape? Or the motel? She had always remembered, again only in snippets and in a strangely confused way, that after the rape she had gone to a cheap motel and stayed there for many days—maybe weeks, as she tried to put herself together. She had thought she was drinking there—something she had not done, except for sips, in her life before or after. She had thought maybe she was trying to forget the rape. But now she wondered. Putting the pieces together, which included quite a number of reactions regarding drinking and being not able to function or losing one's mind, it struck her that her colleague must have put something in her drink. This was actually something she had speculated about before, but now a lot of things fell into place. This is why she could not think straight and could not get it together to leave. And why she was stumbling up the steps—she was being taken somewhere, still woozy. Following these sessions, there were a set of reactions of being scared coming to my office, feeling that she would be in trouble or was being followed. These were also completely out of character for Joyce.

The reactions Joyce was having at this time were a good example of how, as zero process memories fully emerge as experiences, they can make a person seem and feel psychotic. Joyce generally could pull herself together and realize that these must be some kind of reliving, but at times she would be completely taken over by the experiences, and would behave in what would seem like a paranoid manner. She had another anxiety response triggered by a connection to what we were more and more thinking was an experience of being held hostage after the rape. Joyce developed pains in her wrists and ankles, and then she developed red marks and swellings which were quite visible and painful, but short lived. It became clear why she had trouble sleeping—it was like being in the bed where she had been held tied up and drugged for so long. But Joyce was observant enough to realize that this sort of triggering had not been happening previously. She had been able to sleep in beds, and do so many other things by which she was now triggered. But we always knew that she actually had to indulge in certain ideas or fantasies which seemed to defy explanation, until now, in order to be able to fall asleep.

Without going into the details, I can say that they related directly to her situation just as she was escaping from the entrapment. In many other ways, for instance in phobic avoidances of the type of work that she had been engaged in when the rape had happened, she had managed to keep the whole thing very much in the distance, as a vague and veiled memory.

Joyce realized that she had been tied up when she had been held hostage. What made it all make sense is realizing that she had been drugged throughout the time she had been held. She actually had not been drinking in the motel where she stayed after she escaped. She had been recovering from the drugs, first from the direct effects, and then the withdrawal effects. She had assumed the drinking as a story she told herself as she thought of how "out of it" she had been in the motel. Now she knew what that was caused by. Over many sessions and many months, this material emerged, in tiny pieces, strewn all over the place. But then, like a big jigsaw puzzle, all of a sudden we would get a sense of the big picture and all the pieces that we had been gathering had a place in this picture. Often the picture would form when Joyce had one of her more intense relivings, which brought a larger chunk of her past into the present.

At the beginning of one session when I go to get Joyce from the waiting room she looks quite wild, not in the least like herself. I ask her about this. She recounts a memory that she has always had, but not thought about. She remembers looking into the mirror at the motel after the rape, and not recognizing herself. Her hair was all matted and tangled, and her face looked strange, like a scared animal. Now she finally knew why—this was her after being held captive, tied down and drugged for weeks. She says she has looked in the mirror lately, and has seen not herself as she is now, but that girl with the wild hair. This was the beginning of many sessions where we talked about and to that girl—a girl in her early 20s, frightened and abandoned. She had seen this girl in the mirror at other times as well, but was frightened of her, and tried to keep her away. The memories of instances of seeing the girl in the mirror had never been repressed, just avoided and never talked about. The girl contained the memories and feelings of the captivity. She was completely alone and abandoned. I will give a few excerpts from my notes from sessions following this one, and then discuss the connection to splitting of the identity.

Joyce comes into a session and says, "I felt overwhelming anger and rage. I didn't think I could be that angry." She says it was at her husband, but has a feeling that the strength of it is all out of proportion, and must come from the experiences in her 20s. She was woken up many times by dreams, nightmares really, "which is unusual for me. I don't usually have nightmares. It was of being in hospital beds, with I.V.s in me, tied up to the bed. And running and being chased"

"Do you have a sense by whom?"

"No, I don't know who it was."

We talk back and forth, how it might have been a number of people, or one. "You still don't remember how you got away, and I wonder if these dreams are representations of some of that." "I don't know how it ended. I don't know how I got away." I point out that the anger and rage may give us a clue. That she may have had to mobilize that to get away, and put it away to not go back to fight, but rather run away. She disagrees with this last part, feeling that she was in too much danger and would not have been tempted to stay and fight. I bring up how she confronted her abuser in childhood and sent him away. She gets thoughtful and notes that she only started mistrusting people after all this happened in her 20s. Before that she trusted people. She gives examples of how she could stand up to people, but would still generally trust them. I say that maybe after this, she stopped trusting herself, to be able to protect herself, and that from this, she had to be wary of others and could not trust them. Joyce says her relationship with herself was what was destroyed after the rape. She didn't trust herself, maybe to some extent didn't even like herself, afterwards. She begins a deep sobbing, which goes on for a number of minutes. She stops and apologizes, and then continues. It seems not destructive or alarming. But she is very distressed. She stops near the end. "I could have cried for longer if I didn't have to stop. It felt like I was integrating, like parts of me were coming together. But it was very painful. I don't think I've cried like that in here before." She was right.

This session was after we had talked of the wild girl. Talking of her brought up memories and feelings from that time. We had been talking of the issue of how Joyce's relationship with herself had been destroyed. She came to hate this other girl, the girl with the matted hair. It seemed to me that the hatred kept the other girl at a distance. She had in previous sessions become quite angry when I had brought up the other her, the young girl, and when I had sometimes asked her to talk and tell us something. Joyce would flash a withering look, almost of hatred, at me. This would come on quite suddenly and was completely out of keeping with her usual behaviour towards me, even when I had confronted her with things that were difficult for her to bear. She had previously had little trouble being assertive, and even angry with me, but it had not had this quality of rawness and intensity. It is this type of angry response, I have argued, that is a sign of the breakdown of a counterforce defense and the setting up of negative transferences as a defense against uncovering repressed material.

Again, it is not one observation but many, and not many of one type such as the burst of anger at interpretation of the defense, but also observations of different phenomena related to the defense, that I think is convincing regarding the self/self separation and alter formation in DID and in splitting of the identity in general, being a product of powerful counterforce defenses. These other phenomena include the natural history of the split identity formation, and the intense hate that could be mobilized between the identities, that seemed to play an important part in keeping them separate, since as Joyce felt more empathy for the other part of her, the separation between her parts started to dissolve. Later, we realized we have not been seeing the situation clearly, and that there was another alter, a caretaking one, from the time of being confused and overwhelmed taking care of herself in the motel. She had trouble eating, sleeping, and defecating. The caretaking alter was overwhelmed and panicked as she tried desperately to deal with the serious physical symptoms. She and the wild-haired young woman were angry at each other, for specific reasons, but change took place as I interpreted the use of this anger to keep the alters separate, and the use of this separation to keep parts of the traumas hidden. As these alters felt empathy for each other and she for both of them, further integration took place. There were also other uses of splitting of the identity without independent alter formation – something I will discuss in chapter five.

Next session: She says she made a stop at the library, and ran into a metal bench full force– right after she had felt so good, having had a great massage. She fell to the ground, bruised and bleeding. She thought right away when it happened that she should tell me about it, because it seemed related to the reliving of what had happened with her kidnapping. But then things kept going wrong and she got in a worse mood. A feeling takes over in the session, and she says, "I don't know what I'm doing here! This is not like before. I can't stabilize myself. I don't want to relive this." At this point she is fighting me quite strongly, seeming angry at me, saying that she has a nice family and a perfectly good life, and she's going tonight to play cards with her family, and why does she have to relive this? To be overwhelmed and feel awful? She insists this time is different, that it's beyond her capabilities to remember it and relive it. And that she just doesn't want to do it. She implies that she wants to leave right now, that I'm pushing her to do something that's not good for her. She is crying deeply and is very upset, and this goes on for a while. "This is different than the other times. I can't do it. I can't stand it!"

During this time I actually don't feel that she will leave, and don't myself feel tense. I say that she must be reliving what it was like as she struggled to escape her captors: her fear, her anger at them. And also, this shows the sorts of things she was going through as she struggled and as she escaped and ran away. The reliving is very powerful, but I feel reasonably certain that we'll get through it. She talks about how she felt both of her wrists were hurting and a place in one of her wrists began to bleed this day, which made her think of the shape she was in as she escaped. "I fought my way free – I fought someone." What goes through my mind is, did she hurt someone, and perhaps even have to kill someone? What seems especially to turn the tide is when she talks again about looking forward to the card game with her family, and how now she's going to be so upset she may not be able to enjoy it, and I say that that must've been how she felt as she escaped; that she was overwhelmed, completely discombobulated, but that it was the thought of her family, her mother and father, that especially saved her. She says she had thought of killing herself back then when she escaped but the thought of her family drew her forward in time and back home. That thought stopped her from driving into the truck as she was driving away from where she was held captive. "It was also because of what it would've done to the driver, to have to live with that." Then she says after a short pause, "it was a long time." "That you were held hostage, or the time in the motel?" "Both. I must've been so hurt, filled with drugs and bruised, maybe hardly able to walk." She talks of other things related to being hurt, and cries in a way that again feels integrative. (One thing I would draw attention to here, is that Joyce comes up with semantic memories—knowledge memories—for things related to which she has no access to through episodic memories, in this case about how long she had been held captive, and stayed recovering at the motel. This is quite often the case with trauma. These semantic memories can be mistaken by the therapist for speculations, but they are actually a form of memory from the trauma as reliable, and as subject to distortion, being used as screens, etc., as episodic memories. They need to be treated as such, rather than as simple speculations.)

These sessions hopefully give a bit of a sense of how the material emerged and how we dealt with it. The bigger picture was that when Joyce escaped and went to the motel, she tried to rewrite her story. The idea that she had been drunk rather than drugged was part of this rewrite. Some of the memories were pushed to the very early abuse—climbing up the steps, being held hostage in a place and raped. As she remembered being tied up in bed and looking at the ceiling, she connected it to being on her back and looking at the sky in her memory of being raped by her colleague. A number of the details of what she remembered from that rape turned out to be also screens for what happened after. This multiple screening is typical of repression.

But why did Joyce not use splitting of the identity and repression to the same extent in her childhood trauma? It's not that there were not repressions, especially of the time when she was so overwhelmed early in the childhood abuse, but clearly it was not as complete. And the identity splits, which I have come to believe are always present in serious trauma (even if true alters are not) were also present but not so powerfully separated nor so easily delineated as in her adult trauma. I would think one part of it had to do with her complete helplessness and complete feeling of abandonment in the adult situation. She certainly had that at the start of the abuse in childhood, and she repressed that ongoing trauma. But then she managed to control her mind, and use dissociation and compartmentalization flexibly and effectively, both during the abuse and during the rest of her day. This also allowed her to make use of her loving and supportive mother while separating off her anger at her from this loving image. In the adult trauma the use of drugs, most likely some types of tranquilizers, took away her mental ability to do this, while being tied up meant there was no relief or escape from the situation. Joyce's confidence in her ability to keep herself safe, and at the very least to keep her thoughts and mind free, was shattered. When we were analyzing her childhood abuse Joyce said, "I felt they could never take my mind and thoughts from me, no matter what they did to my body, and that's how I survived." It was the extreme helplessness of the adult trauma, with a powerful and realistic fear, even a realistic certainty, that her captors would in the end kill her, that I think led to Joyce's more marked splitting of identity leading to true alters.

Strange and bizarre and life threatening abuse or other traumas are almost always present in the causation of DID. This seems to predispose to not just splitting of the identity, which is there in all severe traumas, but the evolution of this to alter formation, with more elaboration of the split-off identity, and a stronger counterforce defense between the identities. It may be that the extreme terror caused by the imminent death leads to a stronger zero process drive, necessitating stronger counterforces in splitting the identities and with this, the identities take the next step to full independence and further elaboration, as compared to the split-off identities in "regular" severe traumas, which remain rather static and not much elaborated.

As our work continued, Joyce started to feel sorry for the young woman, the other her, and started to feel more connected to her. We saw that the narcissistic men who had always had an attraction for her were related not just or mainly to her early childhood abuser, but rather to the colleague who had raped her and held her hostage in her 20s. She realized that they had many characteristics in common with him, and that this similarity would set strong and until now incomprehensible reactions going in her. She began to integrate and change at a deeper level. I think Joyce's case is useful in looking at the dynamics of splitting of the identity because she was an adult when she instituted the split, and we could follow the process rather closely in our reconstruction of what had happened. One of the main effects of splitting of the identity, whether full alters are formed or not, is a disturbance in the person's relationship with themselves. Some of the techniques used in DID treatment, especially some level of suggestion in calling on the identities, and working on the relationship between the different parts, are useful, in fact I think they are necessary, in analyzing identity splitting. I will discuss these techniques in chapter five.

With these observations and thoughts we reach the formulation that splitting of the identity is what repression looks like in the zero process. Regular repression operates from the outside *upon* zero process memories and drives, and other dynamics that have become entangled with them. While there is usually extensive repression *of* the traumatic drive and memories, splitting of the identity is what repression looks like when it operates *within and between* these memories. We can extend this idea. While avoidance and denial and suppression are directed *at* zero process memories dissociation, zero process denial, and temporal shifting are what these attentional maneuvers look like when operating *within and between* these memories. They are zero process attentional defenses, just as splitting of the identity is a zero process counterforce defense.

In this section I was concentrating on delineating and illustrating the actual mechanisms of identity splitting, using the example of Joyce. Her trauma was unbearable before this maneuver, but the combination of splitting of the identity, alter formation, and repression allowed her to live her adult life after the trauma without too much encumbrance from it, although circumscribed by phobic avoidances and negative relationships that were related to it. It was when these avoidances were seriously challenged by circumstances in her life, that she came back for her second course of therapy, which allowed her to finally become whole again.

Having laid out the basic nature of the zero process and of post-traumatic zero process dynamics, the rest of this book will be concerned with two important applications of these ideas: to an understanding of borderline disorders in the chapter that follows, and to the understanding and development of techniques of trauma therapy in the next one.

The Relation of Borderline Disorders to Trauma

The dynamics of borderline disorders are quite striking, in their effects on others as well as in their intensity. Attempts to comprehend them have led to much innovation in psychoanalytic theory, particularly the concept of projective identification and related dynamics. Let's start with an example from literature, which demonstrates these dynamics as well as any material from a patient. The interaction is from the beginning of Shakespeare's play, King Lear:

Lear:	... . Now, our joy,
	Although our last and least, to whose young love
	The vines of France and milk of Burgundy
	Strive to be interess'd, what can you say to draw
	A third more opulent than your sisters? Speak.
Cordelia:	Nothing, my lord.
Lear:	Nothing?
Cordelia:	Nothing.
Lear:	Nothing will come of nothing. Speak again.
Cordelia:	Unhappy that I am, I cannot heave
	My heart into my mouth. I love your Majesty
	According to my bond; no more nor less.
Lear:	How, now, Cordelia? Mend your speech a little,
	Lest you may mar your fortunes.
Cordelia:	Good my lord,
	You have begot me, bred me, loved me; I
	Return these duties back as are right fit,
	Obey you, love you, and most honour you,
	Why have my sisters husbands, if they say
	They love you all? Happily when I shall wed,
	That lord whose hand shall take my plight shall carry
	Half my love with him, half my care and duty.
	Sure I shall never marry like my sisters,
	To love my father all.

DOI: 10.4324/9781003283218-5

Lear:	But goes thy heart with this?
Cordelia:	Aye, my good lord.
Lear:	So young, and so untender?
Cordelia:	So young, my lord, and true.
Lear:	Let it be so! Thy truth then be thy dower!
	For, by the sacred radiance of the sun,
	The mysteries of Hecate and the night;
	By all the operation of the orbs
	From whom we exist and cease to be;
	Here I disclaim all my paternal care,
	Propinquity and property of blood,
	And as a stranger to my heart and me
	Hold thee from this for ever. The barbarous Scythian,
	Or he that makes his generation messes
	To gorge his appetite, shall to my bosom
	Be as well neighboured, pitied, and relieved,
	As thou my sometime daughter.
King Lear:	Act 1, Scene i

This highly charged interchange between King Lear and his beloved youngest daughter Cordelia begins the play and sets its tragic events in motion. Lear has gathered his court, and his three daughters. "Meantime we shall express our darker purpose," he says. The "darker" means "more obscure" or "secret," but could have other connotations. It turns out that Lear's purpose is to tell them of what could be called his retirement plans: he will divide up his kingdom between the three daughters, and only asks that he be allowed to keep a hundred of his men and be put up alternately in the castle of each daughter. But first, he wants them to declare, "which of you shall we say doth love us most?" This, perhaps predictably, brings trouble. The two older daughters, Goneril and Regan, wax eloquently, or at least verbosely, upon the extent of their love for the old man. As one can gather from what Cordelia says, they essentially claim that their love is boundless, and not constrained or limited by their love for others such as their husbands. Cordelia claims the opposite, and thus the action begins.

There is much to be said about even this small part of this beautifully complex and many layered play. It serves as an introduction to the topic of this chapter, and as a touchstone to which we can return as we discuss key issues related to borderline disorders. Not to say that Lear suffers from a borderline disorder. He is, first of all, a fictional figure. To the extent that he highlights psychological character problems, most commentators see him as self centered, made so perhaps by long exercise of absolute power. In any case, let's start with concrete details. Lear is looking for appeasement and a bowing to his will, and when he does not get it, he does not merely get angry, but becomes enraged, and lashes out in a manner that is clearly out of all proportion to what has happened, as seen by the shocked reaction of the other characters who witness it. Certainly Cordelia has been blunt with him. She has told him something he does not want to hear, and she has done it in front of the whole court, without taking into consideration the touchiness of her father and the humiliation he might feel. His reaction is volcanic. Along with the rage, there is an abrupt flip in Lear's view of Cordelia. She was his most beloved ("our joy/Although our last and least"), and he was very tender to her, promising her "a third more opulent than your sisters," and then suddenly she is so detested that he equates her with those who eat their own children ("he that makes his generation messes/To gorge his appetite.")

For therapists, this is a not unfamiliar reaction. A patient may be in an extremely positive mood towards them. The therapist will feel the pull to get caught up in the elated feeling, related to how well the work is going. The patient will be especially receptive to the therapist. But then all of a sudden, often triggered by a comment, they have a Lear-like reaction. A storm comes. From being loved and idealized, in an instant one becomes derided and demonized. Let me give a brief example of such an inter-action with a young adult patient of mine: L was going through one of her periods of being extremely positive in the analysis, during which she would be receptive to any comments I made, would bring up her own material, and would seem quite excited about what we were doing. This feeling would gallop along over a number of sessions until there was a charged, sexualized excitement in the room. I would feel that we were getting to a real breakthrough, and that I was quite a skilled and brilliant – not to mention charismatic and attractive – analyst. This always ended badly. In this example L talked of anxiety she felt after getting an injection, and how it had reached panic proportions when she was waiting for the subway on her way to my office. She had been talking in previous sessions of her sexual anxieties about penetration. Following this lead, I wondered if there was a sexual meaning to her anxiety about the needles and the subway, especially since she had said that what led to the panic were specifically needles put into a vein, not those into a muscle. The atmo-sphere in the room changed dramatically. Even though she was on the couch, I felt I could see L's face clouding over. There was a very loud and tense silence, and then L spoke. "Why do you say that? I wasn't talking about sex! You're always bringing that up! You're reading way too much into things and not listening to what I'm really upset about!"

The reader may suspect that L was on to something here. Perhaps as a Freudian analyst I was prematurely and crudely making a sexual inter-pretation. This is certainly how I felt as she reacted in anger to my com-ment. When I try to remember more carefully the sequence of what happened in my own mind, I was at first confused and shaken. In fact even though I put these descriptors on this first reaction, I do not remember it very well, except that there was a break in the continuity of my experience. We will return to this aspect of the way in which these interchanges are initiated in the section at the end of this chapter, on projective identification. I think this initial reaction is best referred to as the induction phase of projective identification, to connect it with the similar induction phase at the beginning of hypnosis, where the person's sense of reality and orientation are shaken up, as a prelude to the more stable regressed state of being under hypnosis, which is analogous to the state of deposition of something into the mind of the other in projective identification.

After this brief initiation, I was well and truly under the spell of L's feelings about me, although they were not presented as feelings, but as a reality to which she was having powerful emotional reactions. I was reading too much into things, she said. This quickly became a more general accusation that I did not care for her, did not listen carefully to what she said, and in fact was quite cruel to her. These were not just complaints about a specific action of mine, but general accusations about how I always was. When I wondered about how she had had such a different view of me just prior, she brushed this aside. She clearly remembered what I was talking about but it seemed to have no importance now, and she implied that maybe she was just saying those positive things about me to please me. L kept on talking about how insensitive I was, building to a crescendo of accusation in which I was pictured as the worst of sadists. I said that I had merely been following up on her statements about her sexual anxieties from the previous session. This really made her blood boil. "Now you're just trying to blame me even more!" she exclaimed. These sorts of interactions continued throughout this session and the next.

No reaction on my part, whether explanatory, conciliatory, interpretive, or supportive (and I certainly tried them all) could stem or contain the storm of anger and hurt feelings. If I could have taken a step back as all this was going on it would have been obvious that the affective storm, and the image of me that was getting worse by the minute, had a reality and a momentum all their own, quite uninfluenced by what I said, or by any other aspect of reality for that matter. This sort of implacable affect storm is what King Lear displays in the passage quoted. It blows in like a hurricane, and nothing can slow it down, until it blows itself out. After a number of days, my patient L had calmed down somewhat, and after a number of weeks, the storm had largely passed. At a certain point, L became more positive, but seemed not to appreciate the stark changes in her mood and her view of me that had taken place. When I brought this up, she did remember, but was both a little embarrassed by the memory, and tended to brush it aside, as being of little interest to her, just as she had previously brushed aside my comments about her positive view of our relationship when the storm was in full force. Like the landscape after a hurricane, I was left quite shaken even after the winds and rain had passed.

There are several things in what I have described, both in my patient L and in King Lear, that are characteristic of those suffering from borderline personality disorder. These include the affect storms, the split image of others as either all good or all bad, a very strong tendency to project out the internal world into the external one, and the induction of powerful responses in others related to these projections. While these and a number of other characteristics are distinctive, it is important to emphasize that they exist along a spectrum of severity, with the psychiatric designation "borderline personality disorder" of various classification systems only capturing the more severe end, and also that almost everyone can display some of these dynamics at times. In this chapter I will refer to borderline disorders or borderline characteristics, with the understanding that the actual presentation in any person may vary quite a bit. Also, I believe specific borderline characteristics and deficits vary relatively independently from many other psychological characteristics, so that those with borderline difficulties may be more obsessional, or have more of a tendency to use repression like a classic hysteric; they may tend generally to externalize, such as Lear and my patient L, or they may tend more towards internalization and thus have their emotional explosions more quietly and internally; they may be more narcissistic or less so. This is not to say that the specific borderline deficits may not affect each of these characteristics (such as narcissism or the functioning of repression, for example), but this does not preclude these and many other factors varying quite a bit from one person with borderline features to another.

With these caveats, I will try in this chapter to delve into some aspects borderline disorders. This is a large topic, about which much has been written. I have limited my discussion to those areas where the theory of trauma and the zero process intersects with that of borderline disorders. These points of intersection form the topics of each of the following sections. The overarching theme is the disentanglement of trauma from borderline disorders. As there is much in the prevailing ideas about borderline disorders that tends towards this entanglement, I will be taking issue with some widely accepted ideas about the nature and causation of these disorders. In the first section I will contrast borderline disorders as exemplars of the intrusion of the primary process into the ego, with posttraumatic states, in which the zero process intrudes. The next section, on the causation and dynamics of borderline disorders, will discuss developmental trauma. This is seen by many as a key causative factor in borderline disorders. I will suggest that the central feature in those with borderline disorders is a difficulty stabilizing libidinal investment in themselves and others—the causation for this being both heredity and certain types of developmental interference and traumas. In other words, trauma is not the central cause of borderline disorders, and this is why they look so different from post-traumatic disorders. But then what is the relationship between the two? This is explored in the next section, which especially looks at the reasons for the susceptibility of borderlines to being easily traumatized and their quite distinctive post-traumatic effects. The last section, on projective identification, looks at projective identification as a specific counterforce defense against drives within the primary process, in people with weak repressions, and contrasts this with both identification with the aggressor, and with splitting of the identity, which is the specific counterforce defense within the zero process. Projective identification is discussed as a common psychological underpinning for many forms of abuse.

The Zero Process, the Primary Process, and the Secondary Process Revisited

Freud first presented his ideas about the primary process in his major work on dreams (1900). It is quite striking, and I think a piece of evidence for the validity of Freud's formulations, that the characteristics that he described regarding the primary process are so clearly in evidence in borderline disorders, even though Freud developed these ideas in relation to quite different material—the analysis of dreams and neuroses. In fact, the discovery of borderline disorders as a separate category was only made at the end of Freud's life, and was not known to him. I will describe a bit of this history in the next section, but at this point would like to dive right in to the nature of borderline disorders, and their striking similarity to Freud's characterization of the primary process.

Freud described how in the primary process various seemingly contradictory trends, such as love and hate towards the same person, existed happily side by side, with no conflict or attempt to find a middle ground. We can see something similar in the sudden switch in the image of the other shown by Lear and my patient L. If one looked at just these single incidents, one might think it was merely a case of an angry, defensive response, which of course then coloured the image of the person, whether my image in the mind of my patient or Cordelia's in Lear's mind. But the sudden switch and the extremes in terms of the loved and hated images are clues that something else is at work. In the case of my patient the history of these kinds of switches suggested that there were certainly two very different images of me, and also of others, and two very different sets of feelings associated with the images. The key thing is that these did not come into conflict with each other but rather simply popped up sequentially. When I reminded L of her previously quite opposite feelings towards me, she remembered it vaguely. It was not repressed, but she dismissed it with a psychical wave of the mind, as of no consequence. This is a common response among borderlines.

Because in borderlines primary process characteristics have invaded the ego, we are able to see them and even hear words being put on them. It is as if the primary process could speak, when L says she knows that she had a good image of me, but it's not so important. She is giving voice to the lack of connection of one attitude, thought, or feeling with another, the lack of interest of each in the other, one might say, that characterizes the contents of the primary process. This lack of synthesis is the well known "splitting" of borderline disorders, usually seen as one of their defining character-istics. I remember first being shown this in a psychiatric clinical rotation in medical school. The staff were going over the inpatients with each other in the morning rounds, and one of them was well liked by one member of the staff, who felt she was really trying her best, but was seen as manipulative and not to be trusted by one of the other staff members. One of the psy-chiatrists pointed out to me that this was common in, even diagnostic of, borderline disorders—the staff would themselves "split" in their attitude towards the patient. This manifestation of splitting demonstrates another key aspect of borderline dynamics—the very strong tendency for internal battles and characteristics to manifest externally, in others. This mirrors the lack of firm self/other and self/world boundaries in the primary process.

Borderline parents will often split their children, in the sense that they will see one as bad, and another as good but also, in that they will often set them fighting one against the other much like the staff in the hospital did. It is probably not a stretch to see the strife between Lear's daughters as something akin to this. (This may also bring to the reader's mind certain politicians and public figures who have this effect, sometimes on whole nations or even more broadly.) This type of splitting is one of the many ways in which the inner world of the borderline plays out in the wider world, with different people taking on different parts of the per-son's inner world. This splitting is clearly not just a passive lack of synthesis, but involves active moves on the part of the person to bring it about. In fact, internal splitting in borderline disorders is usually con-ceptualized as a largely active process of keeping different trends, such as love and hate, apart—for instance by Melanie Klein (1945, 1946, 1958) and most Kleinian authors who followed her, such as Bion (1959). Klein herself worked with very disturbed borderline and psychotic children, and from this work developed her ideas of active splitting of various images, such as the bad breast and the good breast, beginning almost from birth. This splitting was seen as motivated by anxieties such as fear of destroying the good breast and the need to protect it from the infant's death instinct.

Other authors as well (for instance Kernberg, 1967) talk of active splitting in the case of borderline disorders. One of the proofs of this is that when one tries to bring the different split aspects together, in the face of their indifference, the person will get anxious. If the split was simply due to a lack of synthesis, this reaction would be hard to explain. However, I don't think this argues against the point that I am trying to make. I am certainly not saying that in the borderline condition, what we see is pure id functioning, or pure primary process functioning. Rather, the regular functioning of the ego, which manages such things as contact with reality and defenses, is invaded to a greater extent than normal by aspects of primary process functioning. One of these is the aforementioned lack of synthesis, which once it is present in the ego, is of course used for defensive purposes—especially so since selective repression, which usually does the heavy lifting in keeping drives in check, is weakened. I will discuss this aspect later, but let's continue with the primary process, and see what else it can explain about borderline conditions.

Freud described the easy mobility of the investment in the primary process, leading to the displacements and condensations seen in dreams. In borderline dynamics, one is often caught off guard by the strong reactions to what one would think are relatively minor occurrences or interventions of the therapist, or comments by friends and relatives. In those instances where one can retrospectively gain insight into what brought the reaction on, the freewheeling displacement and condensation of interest from something that would be important to other things is seen to be the culprit. And speaking of the strong reactions, these too—that is, a lack of modulation and inhibition of drives and affects—are characteristic of the primary process. It is the secondary process that adds inhibition, modulation, and the reality principle. Freud talked of the secondary process as coming about through the "binding" of the energy that moves about so freely in the primary process. Borderlines are classically described as displaying a "stable instability"—that is, they can be counted on to not stabilize for too long in one attitude or emotion. "Stable instability" is also a good description of the situation in the primary process.

Freud (1900) noted that in the primary process, no distinction was made between fantasies and reality. For the borderline as well, this distinction can vanish at times, especially in situations of high feeling. There was some evidence that L was experiencing the emergence of sadomasochistic sexual fantasies when she felt intense anxiety on getting a needle, and being in the subway, both of which were symbolic of aspects of these conflicted fantasies and wishes. When I wondered about a possible sexual meaning of the anxieties, L not only got defensive, but became convinced that I was being sadistic towards her. And not just in that instance, but more generally. I was a sadistic and mean person, who had been so even in previous times when she had originally believed that I was nice and helpful. Here not only the lack of distinction between fantasy and reality but also the high reactivity, the splitting of basic feelings and drives, and the lack of firm distinction between self and other were all in evidence.

Freud said that in the primary process there is no negation. Things simply are. There is no possibility that they may not exist or may not be true. Similarly, borderlines evince a certainty beyond mere confidence in many of their pronouncements—even or especially the ones based on projection and confusion of fantasy and reality. This has a compelling effect on those around them, who often cannot help but believe these pronouncements at least emotionally, even when they are aware that they are not true. (Here too the reader may find themselves thinking of various leaders throughout history, up to the turmoiled present, who have had this effect on people.) I was shaken not just by the strength of L's accusation, but by the feeling that I really had been sadistic, and was perhaps torturing L with my interpretations, and enjoying it. The confusion between fantasy and reality, and the lack of negation, can create quite a disconcerting effect. The borderline can seem at times psychotic—for instance when they insist, and are quite sure, that you shouted at them, even though you did no such thing. And yet they are not clinically psychotic. They are quite capable of testing and knowing reality, and of thinking rationally. These basic functions—one could call them the basic machinery of the mind that does such things as thinking—are intact, as they are not intact in a psychotic process such as schizophrenia.

Ideally, I would at this point compare the difficulties with reality in borderline disorders to those in different forms of psychosis—but this would take us too far afield. Ideally I would also compare the invasion of regular functioning by the primary process in borderline disorders to a different mixing up of the ego and id in obsessionality. Here the ego remains very much intact, as do self/other differentiation, repressions, etc., and yet classic obsessional dynamics also involve such things as the thinking processes taking on primary process qualities. The striking similarities and just as striking differences between these two dynamics can, I think, be briefly described by the formula that in borderline dynamics a weak ego is invaded by primary process functioning, while in obsessional dynamics, the id and the primary process are invaded by an overly strong ego and secondary process. But this statement is just the beginning of a deeper comparison. These sorts of comparative studies have been done—more so those comparing borderline and psychotic disorders than the in some ways more fascinating and theoretically important comparison of borderline and obsessional disorders and dynamics. I hope to present some thoughts on the latter comparison in my next book, as it is fruitful in approaching both individual and social development, but at this point I will proceed to my main point in bringing all this up: a comparison of the primary process aspects of borderline disorders to the zero process aspects of post-traumatic disorders.

In chapter two I compared the primary process and the zero process. In each of the characteristics described, I believe that the core characteristics of borderline disorders are those of the primary process. I noted that in the primary process fantasies are confused with present reality, which describes also the situation in borderline disorders. In the zero process present reality is confused with specific past unprocessed traumatic realties. However, one theory of what is going on in such situations as my patient L feeling unloved and attacked is that a past trauma of maltreatment, perhaps from very early in her infancy or childhood, was triggered by something in the therapy and things I had done, so that she was in fact confusing the present reality with a past reality of developmental trauma. There was in fact no evidence that early traumas of neglect and/or maltreatment had taken place for L. There were incidents of misunderstanding and conflicts later in childhood but these seemed to be not so severe—although her reactions were. Those who support the idea of the importance of early trauma may suggest that I had not gone deeply enough. This is certainly possible. Also, a single case cannot be used as evidence for more general causation.

The basic idea outlined above, that in fact what I am claiming is a primary process confusion of fantasy and wish with reality is the living out of actual early developmental trauma, and that this early trauma is the main, or at least one of the main, causative factors in borderline disorders, is a view widely held among psychodynamic theorists. The more specific interpretation is that the interaction between patient and therapist is a replay of what happened at a very young age between infant and caregiver, that the therapist's reactions within this interaction (such as mine of making the sexual interpretation and then feeling like a sadist) contain clues about this early interaction, and that this early set of interactions are causative of borderline problems. This is a complex area of theorizing in relation to borderline dynamics, and I will approach it from a number of angles. Here I will do so from the perspective of the zero process. In the following sections, I will look at other aspects.

It is important to clarify what we are really referring to in discussing the reactions of borderline patients. This net can be thrown too widely. After all, borderlines also will have traumas, and thus will have the confusion between the past reality of the trauma and present reality—a hallmark of the zero process—pop up at times. I am not arguing against the presence or connection to traumas of such reactions. These types of post-traumatic reactions are present in both those suffering from borderline disorders and those who are not. But there are the reactions characteristic of, and specific to, borderline conditions, such as the examples that I have given, that involve a split (good and bad) image of the other person, and usually a very specific charge against the other person, that they do not care enough, that they are mean, and that they are intentionally sadistic. The other side of this reaction, also demonstrated in the two brief examples given, is the extremely positive and idealizing view of the other. It is this very characteristic set of reactions that I would argue are a product of, and representation of, the workings of the primary process, specifically the lack of synthesis between differing emotional and drive trends in a person.

One piece of evidence for this is that these specific reactions do not have some of the defining characteristics of the zero process, which would mark them out as the product of trauma. The specific dissociated zero process memories from trauma are evoked by present concrete details that link to the trauma, and this leads to reliving, and a confusion of past trauma with present reality. The reality is rigidly maintained and repeated. As an example of being uncaring as part of a post-traumatic reaction displaying the characteristics of the zero process, we might look back to Joyce, and her reliving of her rape and abuse during her captivity, described at the beginning of chapter two. When the reliving of the trauma was in full swing, Joyce felt I was attacking her, as her rapist had done. The reactions were quite concrete and specific, and repeated each time they were triggered, with many of the same perceptions and body feelings, although new details did emerge over time. By contrast, the classic borderline reaction involves a changing set of accusations—you didn't listen last time they were talking, and seemed to be making fun of them, or something else the next time—centered around the specific accusation of not loving them enough, and not being invested in them more generally.

I believe that the accusation of not caring enough relates to a specific difficulty that the borderline themselves has that is at the heart of the disorder, and that is externalized. This aspect I will discuss in the next section, just below. But for now, I would like to emphasize the primary process characteristics of displacement and condensation, of constant movement and change, in these reactions and accusations. These are characteristics of the primary process and are quite different from the fixed repetition of the memories of the zero process. I realize for some these theoretical considerations may not carry much weight, especially if they do not use the concepts—but my point is to prove the usefulness of this way of looking at things by using the concepts. If we look at situations such as that with my patient L, or the fictional one with King Lear, we see the eruption of powerful feelings and drives, such as the sadomasochistic wishes and conflicts that seemed to be emerging in L's case, and the wish for love and adoration, and anger when this is thwarted, in the case of Lear. While of course the situation with Lear is fictional, it does depict very well the childish and regressed state in which repressions and sublimations break down and feelings and wishes overwhelm the person. Lear asks for protestations of love, and is pleased with his daughters who say they love him best of all, like a little child who wants to be the favourite of his parents and bitterly resents any rivals, whether the other parent or siblings. When his wish for total narcissistic gratification is thwarted Lear's rage, like that of a two year old, knows no bounds.

But let's take up the counter argument against my idea that these borderline reactions are not trauma related. Even though these reactions seem to have drive and primary process characteristics, and look somewhat different than the trauma repetitions of such patients as Peggy and Joyce, this may be due to the fact that in the case of borderline disorders it's not just that the trauma occurred very early, but also was of a specific type—a deficit in caring and warmth, in help in containing and processing feelings, in learning how to recognize and think about one's own and another person's mental states—all these failures repeated chronically and happening at an age when the growth of the self is just starting. Doesn't it make sense that a failure such as this might lead to the various deficits and problems in self image, affect regulation, and basic human relating that we see in borderlines?

My patient Peggy was brought up by a mother with paranoid schizophrenia who was often quite out of touch with reality, talking to delusional figures, at times becoming unpredictably violent, and also sexually abusing Peggy. There were certainly many consequences and effects of all of this, some of which I have already described (such as living in a second reality, of fear and aloneness, all her life), but being left with borderline deficits or dynamics was not one of these consequences. Peggy did not have the tendency to split object or self images, nor to project her own issues onto others, beyond the usual amount, nor the problems with diffusion of identity, that are part of borderline dynamics. She developed a good therapeutic alliance with me, which deepened over time, and throughout her life had strong and deep emotional relationships with others. Her "splits" were between her past traumatic reality, especially the scary early times with a psychotic mother and her mother's sexual abuse of her, and her present reality; they were not between love and hate, or other basic emotions.

A differentiation between the characteristics of the zero process and the primary process may seem a very narrow approach to borderline dynamics, and it is. But sometimes narrowing the view, bringing the details sharply into focus, can allow us to see things we may not see otherwise. In order to avoid misunderstanding, I want to state clearly what I have been trying to establish: I am arguing, using the theory of the zero process, that certain defining aspects of borderline disorder display characteristics of the primary process, and not the zero process. These include borderline splitting of global affects and self and objects, and reality distortion based on confusing wishes and fantasies with reality. These characteristics, signs of overwhelming by internal drives and affects, should be distinguished from dissociation of zero process traumatic memories, and reality distortion based on confusion between these specific memories and present reality—signs of the enduring effects of traumatic environmental overwhelming. In asserting this, I am certainly not asserting that people with borderline difficulties may not also have zero process post-traumatic phenomena, and I am also not asserting that trauma may not play a part in weakening repressions and other ego functions that may exacerbate borderline dynamics. But I *am* asserting that borderline dynamics are not post-traumatic phenomena, and that a careful study of the zero process as compared to the primary process can make this clear. I think borderline disorders have a complex causation, beginning with certain constitutional weaknesses, which interact with environmental factors, including traumas and deficits in caretaking, to lead to the dynamics we call borderline. At this point, the discussion grows beyond the narrow confines of different forms of mental functioning, and we turn in the next section to a broader consideration of borderline disorders.

Dynamics, Deficits, and Development in Borderline Disorders

Borderline disorders were not described or well understood during the early development of psychoanalysis. One of Freud's most famous patients, the "Wolf Man" as he is called because of his wolf dream from when he was four years old (Freud, 1918), clearly had borderline deficits and dynamics from early childhood on, as detailed by Blum (1974). However, Freud diagnosed him as a severe obsessional, while the pre-eminent psychiatrist of the time, Emil Kraepelin, thought he suffered from manic depressive disorder. The conceptual leap of seeing borderline disorder as a separate thing had not yet happened.

Blum (1974) suggests that serious obsessionality in childhood, such as the wolf man suffered from, often covers over or stabilizes a borderline or psychotic structure. He notes borderline children have difficulties in many areas, which are sustained and severe. The young Wolf Man felt people were looking at him, and could not distinguish waking from dreaming for a while after awakening. He would fly into a rage as a child when he thought people were looking at him, and was reclusive and secretive. Blum (2013a) describes how after the wolf dream, the young child became oversensitive to the point of paranoia, screaming that people were looking at him, and being uncontrollable. He had extreme shyness and self consciousness in adolescence. Each of these symptoms and reactions by themselves could be found in a more neurotic child—but it was their strength, persistence, and constant flux (the stable instability of the primary process) that suggests borderline difficulties. They evidence the difficulties in setting up stable selective repressions and other structures and in stabilizing emotional reactions.

In a demonstration of his weak repressions, the Wolf Man began his first session with Freud by calling him a "Jew-swine," and expressing the wish both to defecate on him and to have him penetrate him anally (Blum, 2013a). Freud apparently took this all in stride, and continued with the treatment. The analysis that followed (Freud, 1918) led to discoveries related to early stages of development, to ideas about the "primal scene" where a child views their parents having sex, to further development of the idea of deferred action, and much else. Weak repressions give easier access to early fantasies and wishes than is the case in more neurotic patients, but there are also aspects specific to borderline dynamics mixed in. Freud stressed what he saw as certain constitutional tendencies in the Wolf Man: the intense passivity of his patient, and that he did not give up any developmental position. Blum (2013b) notes that the swaddling of the patient for his first 9 months may have played a part in the passivity. These tendencies and reactions to the swaddling could be seen as illustrative of the interaction of constitution and experience we see in borderlines. Not every baby who is swaddled will develop the wolf man's level of passivity, but it is quite possible that for him the swaddling experience could not be sublimated and otherwise transformed and contained, in the same way as for many others. Why this is so for borderlines I will discuss in the next section, but let's first follow the history of the discovery of these disorders for a bit.

It was just a year before Freud's death that the first clear exposition of the nature of borderline disorders appeared. Stern (1938) described a group of patients who differed in specific ways from neurotic patients. They were touchy, narcissistic, had difficulty forming a therapeutic alliance, and had a very negative reaction to enlightening interpretations. Stern described the feeling of being controlled, which is actually one of the most reliable signs that one is dealing with a borderline disorder. This feeling is especially strong in patients with a narcissistic disorder in the borderline range. Already at this early stage, Stern's (1945) ideas on causation were basically the same as those of the majority of present day authors: he argued that the causation of borderline disorders was traumatic—not acute trauma or sexual abuse but rather ongoing trauma at a very young age which left the ego vulnerable and weak in terms of facing any further upset or trauma. This is what is now usually referred to as developmental trauma. He felt that this early trauma came from the mother's side, and that you could see its effects by the hunger for love and affection of these patients. This is what they did not get from their mother. Although there are no memories retained from this early period, one can infer this early situation by the patient's reactions in therapy, as well as their reactions in relationships more generally.

The key insight of Stern and other early workers was that, despite the name, borderline disorders represented something different from either neurosis, psychosis, or many of the other previously described conditions such as bipolar disorder, or depressive disorders. Because the symptomatology is so changeable and at times matches that of many of these other syndromes there was a tendency to see borderline disorders as simply a worse version, or a different version, of something else. Severe borderline cases were most likely diagnosed as psychotic or manic depressive, while somewhat less severe ones were seen as suffering from a severe neurosis. Today, many see borderline disorders, as did Stern, as a type of post- traumatic disorder, related specifically to chronic early trauma. But if borderline disorders are not any of these, what kind of a disturbance are they, and what defines them, in terms of their deeper dynamics and causation?

Since the early days of its discovery, there has been a lot of work from many different angles—statistical, clinical, etc.,—on delineating the basic characteristics of the borderline spectrum. Through this, it was realized that the confusing nature of the disorder, with its ever changing symptomatology, moods, capacity to test reality, and much else, was actually one of its main defining features. The others included the splitting tendencies and difficulties with reality testing described in the last section, as well as difficulties with impulse control, and with control of affects, so that a sad feeling or an anxious one could very quickly run away on the person and become overwhelming. Even here, though, this running away will happen unpredictably, in keeping with the stable instability that is a hallmark of the disorder. Anxiety and anger at high levels are usually the dominant affects. There is a serious deficit in the capacity to self soothe and a constant dependence on others and/or some exciting situations, drugs, etc. for good feelings, which are threatening to collapse at any moment.

From a psychoanalytic point of view, at a deeper level, the two defining psychological features of borderline personality are identity diffusion and a lack of object constancy. Object constancy refers to the ability to keep a mental representation of the other emotionally invested in one's mind when one is not with them. Intellectual knowledge of the other person may be intact. What is deficient is a stable emotional investment. This makes the borderline dependent on the actual presence of the person for reassurance, and makes them prone to severe abandonment anxiety, and feelings of emptiness and aloneness that are of a different order than those of more neurotic individuals. Identity diffusion is simply the playing out of this same difficulty in relation to the self image or self representation. In other words, the person cannot maintain a stable emotional investment in their own sense of themselves, so that the self image and identity are ever changing and never stable. I believe that the deepest conceptualization of all this is that there is a deficit in the ability to stabilize libidinal investment in the self and in others. Many borderline phenomena are a consequence of this basic difficulty. These include the difficulty with self/other boundaries and the very powerful tendency to have the internal world play out quite extensively with other people in the external world. I will now describe some of the ideas of others. This will allow us to further elucidate the theory of a basic deficit in libidinal stability and sublimation as causative of borderline disorders by comparing it to these other theories.

The study of borderline disorders has reshaped psychoanalytic theory. Melanie Klein (1945, 1958) analyzed borderline and psychotic children and from this work developed her influential theory about splitting defenses that attempted to keep the "good" object protected from the child's aggression, by splitting it off from the "bad" object that is hated. She described splitting, projective, and introjective mechanisms beginning from very early infancy, driven especially by fear of the death instinct destroying the self or other. The splitting and borderline tendency to project out the inner world into the outer one finds a prominent place in Kleinian theory, as does the constant flux and primary process lack of stability, in ideas about a constant back and forth between the paranoid/schizoid and depressive positions. Otto Kernberg (1967, 1975) developed a theory of splitting which took much from Klein, and also from Edith Jacobson's (1964) ideas about the development of the self and object world. His developmental timetable was more in keeping with ego psychologists such as Jacobson and especially Margaret Mahler (1971, Mahler et al., 1975), in seeing the lack of integration of object images and splitting conflicts taking place in the third and fourth years of life. Kernberg felt that it was especially because of excessively high levels of aggression (he thought mainly constitutional) that the child resisted bringing the good and bad images of the object or the self together in the lead up to the oedipal period. This splitting defense was seen by Kernberg as decisive: it interfered with the development of repression and of more stable internal structures, and the person was thrown back on using defenses such as primitive denial and idealization, along with splitting of self and objects into good and bad. The difficulties in building up inner structure and stabilizing it under this kind of splitting regime leads to weak ego structure and also a lack of proper internalization and development of the superego, which remains immature and harsh.

Despite their many differences, both Kernberg and Klein saw the genesis of borderline disorder as rooted in active defensive processes used to deal with destructive drives. In contrast, Margaret Mahler (1971) realized that specific difficulties in borderline disorders could be related to her discoveries about the process of separation and individuation in the young child, but she tended to see both constitutional factors and the actual behaviour of caretakers as significant to the difficulties in negotiating the separation-individuation process. She traced the timing of major fixation and causation to toddlerhood and later, when the child is fighting for a separate and autonomous sense of self. Failures in this process, she suggested, may be the basis for the emergence of borderline dynamics. Since Mahler studied the development of libidinal object constancy, her work and ideas were directly related to the specific difficulties faced by borderline patients. It is worth stressing again that while the difficulty or deficit that borderlines suffer from is often referred to simply as "object constancy," Mahler's work, and the basic borderline deficit, relate to constancy of the libidinal object. The object as known or seen by the ego is often intact—this object only disappears in severe psychosis. It is the emotional investment in the object that is shaky. The same is true of what is called "identity diffusion"—it is not an ego or intellectual deficit in knowing the self, but a lack of stability in the libidinal investment in the self.

It is beyond the scope of this chapter to cover the voluminous literature of more recent times on borderline disorder. The general trend has been to trace causation, in agreement with Mahler, to a greater extent to external impingements and deprivations, but to push these to very early times, before toddlerhood usually. These ideas about very early causation were much influenced by Klein and those she influenced. To take just one example as a stand-in for many others, we could look at Bion's (1959) well known paper, "Attacks on Linking." A quote from this paper is a good illustration both of the view of early causation and of its inference from adult analytic interactions: "Associations from a period in the analysis earlier than that from which these illustrations have been drawn showed an increasing intensity of emotions in the patient. This originated in what he felt was my refusal to accept parts of his personality. Consequently he strove to force them into me with increased desperation and violence. His behaviour, isolated from the context of the analysis, might have appeared to be an expression of primary aggression. The more violent his phantasies of projective identification, the more frightened he became of me. There were sessions in which such behaviour expressed unprovoked aggression, but I quote this series because it shows the patient in a different light, his violence a reaction to what he felt was my hostile defensiveness. The analytic situation built up in my mind a sense of witnessing an extremely early scene. I felt that the patient had experienced in infancy a mother who dutifully responded to the infant's emotional displays. The dutiful response had in it an element of impatient 'I don't know what's the matter with the child.' My deduction was that in order to understand what the child wanted the mother should have treated the infant's cry as more than a demand for her presence. From the infant's point of view she should have taken into her, and thus experienced, the fear that the child was dying. It was this fear that the child could not contain. He strove to split it off together with the part of the personality in which it lay and project it into the mother.

An understanding mother is able to experience the feeling of dread, that this baby was striving to deal with by projective identification, and yet retain a balanced outlook. This patient had had to deal with a mother who could not tolerate experiencing such feelings and reacted either by denying them ingress, or alternatively by becoming a prey to the anxiety which resulted from introjection of the infant's feelings. The latter reaction must, I think, have been rare: denial was dominant." (pp. 312–313.)

There are many things in this quote that illustrate a basic set of assumptions and ideas related to severe emotional disorders that have grown in popularity, and are dominant today in much of psychoanalytic literature. Bion describes his patient attempting to get him to accept parts of his personality into himself, through projective identification. "The more violent his phantasies of projective identification, the more frightened he became of me," he notes. This fits with a projective identification where as the patient projects his aggression into Bion, the patient becomes scared of him, since now he experiences his aggression as residing in Bion, and threatening him. I would certainly agree with Bion that the patient's aggression is not primary, but defensive. He is scared of Bion. Aggression used as a defense to forcefully put a part of a person into someone else is also an intrinsic part of the defense of projective identification. This aspect of borderline dynamics, including the more interactional view of projective identification that Bion presaged and that has been developed further since his time, will be discussed in detail in a separate section at the end of this chapter. There are two further inferential steps Bion makes in this quote that I will deal with now.

Firstly, Bion infers that what is happening in the sessions is that he is "witnessing an extremely early scene." He feels that he can deduce the nature of the scene in quite a bit of detail. He feels that his patient's mother had misunderstood his crying as merely a call for her presence, when in reality her child was calling for her to take in and contain his fear of dying. Bion states that "An understanding mother is able to experience the feeling of dread, that this baby was striving to deal with by projective identification, and yet retain a balanced outlook." His mother was unable to do this, and thus the patient was left with these feelings, which he tried to get Bion to take in. The idea of this type of interaction in therapy being a consequence of, to some extent a replay of, and also direct evidence for, what happened in the very early relationship with the caregiver, is now almost standard fare. What has generally been added and developed in more recent work is the use of the therapist's countertransference as a guide to what happened in infancy, something only hinted at by Bion.

Bion's second inference, closely connected to the first, is that the mother's inability or unwillingness to help her son by containing his fear of dying was the cause of his later disturbance. This idea is based on a theory that sees the most important influence on, and input into, much of development as being the interaction between the mother and infant. Many key functions, such as thinking, modulation of affects, and the ability to form stable emotional bonds are seen as largely created through this interaction. Most theorists view the outcome of development as involving a complex interplay between inherited tendencies and abilities and environmental inputs and interactions. However modern theory, especially when it comes to causation of borderline and other severe disorders, in practice takes the view that many key mental functions are essentially created by the interaction between mother and child.

Bion is a good example of this kind of theorizing. For instance he saw basic functions such as thinking as created by the mother in her interactions with the infant. My belief is that this collapses a long process of maturation and development down to infancy, even though many of the various aspects of thinking, such as objectivation and abstraction, mature only much later. Along with the temporal collapse, and partly as a consequence of it, this kind of model also sees functions such as thinking as unitary, rather than as complex conglomerates built up over time. This type of theorizing is generally more appealing to common sense, and also often feels more profound, as it is less reductive. But it does not model the complexities of real life very well. In his clinical example, Bion sees the mother as having to contain and process the patient's intense feelings in order for him to be able to do it in the future, and Bion sees her failure to do this as a direct cause of her son's incapacity to do this as an adult.

The view that the deficits in functioning of severe disorders are a product of failures in very early care has a long history in psychoanalysis. Schizophrenia and autism were both seen by many, beginning in the 1950s, as a product of "refrigerator mothers" who lacked all warmth, and thus impaired their child's development of attachment to the human world. There were both observational and theoretical reasons for these ideas. Theoretically, if more severe neurosis was caused by earlier fixations, why would not even more severe disorders be caused by even earlier traumas and deprivations? From the observational side, mothers and fathers of such children often interacted differently with their child. (But this could just as easily be as a consequence of dealing with a very different type of child, than a cause of the child's problems.) There were also the observations on the severe difficulties and developmental arrests suffered by institutionalized and other seriously neglected children, although these disturbances differed in many ways from autism and psychosis—and from borderline personality disorder. Certainly in the case of autism and schizophrenia, although there are psychoanalysts who still adhere to the hypothesis of unempathic parenting, opinion has tilted away from this view, towards hereditary deficits as primary. Just as is the case with autism and schizophrenia, I believe that borderline disorders have been caught up in a powerful tendency to collapse complex chains of causation, and to blame the mother.

These ideas about borderline disorders are treated by many therapists and theoreticians as so firmly established, or so obviously true, that they need no further questioning, but rather are used as a priori assumptions from which to begin to think about a case or build up a theory. In my experience whenever someone presents a case with very deleterious early treatment or deprivation, who nonetheless shows resilience or connects well to the therapist, the presenter or someone in the audience will invariably comment that this must be because they had someone in their early life who connected with them and gave them love. On the other hand if a patient is doing quite badly, with many borderline features, the negative features of early caregivers, such as narcissism, depression, etc., will be highlighted. It has often struck me that there is never an even handed attempt to look at the evidence. Perhaps the borderline patient, along with the somewhat narcissistic mother, also spent a lot of time with her quite warm and loving grandmother—why did this not make a difference? We assume positive influences led to a good outcome in the non-borderline case—why was there no such effect on the borderline one?

Whether constitutional or acquired, different deficits have been proposed as causative of borderline disorders. Fonagy and his co-workers (e.g., Fonagy et al., 2011) have especially suggested a deficit in mentalization—the ability to form models of the person's mind and the minds of others. They believe constitutional factors play a variable part, but that the unvarying factor is a mother who cannot reflect upon, contain, and reflect back to the infant, their own mental state. One difficulty with this view is that borderlines are quite capable of awareness and detailed knowledge of the mental states of others, both when in a not emotionally overwhelmed state, and also when they use this knowledge in inductions of emotion in, and manipulations of, others. Fonagy and his coworkers (e.g., Fonagy et al., 2002) acknowledge this fact, but deal with it by suggesting that while the ability to understand the mental states of others is present, it is often defended against. This is of course a very different dynamic, which to my mind undermines the idea of a deficit in mentalization. As with many of the other popular psychoanalytic theories about the causation and dynamics of borderline disorders, that of Fonagy and his coworkers sees causation as largely resting in deficits in early caregiving (although they acknowledge the influence of constitutional factors more than do many other theorists), leading to some kind of deficit in basic ego capacities, such as mentalization or symbolization.

I think observation fits better with a theory in which these basic ego capacities are preserved, but are impacted at times by a deficit in the ability to neutralize drives consistently and in a stable manner. I see the constitutional factors as the primary, invariant ones, while the relational and other environmental ones such as abuse, traumas, etc. are the variable factors, that interact with the basic deficit in different ways, as they do in autism and schizophrenia. I think there is a partial deficit in the ability to stabilize libidinal investment in others, in the self, and in the world more generally. There seems also to be a corresponding difficulty in properly neutralizing aggression in order to use it for structure building (repression, self/other boundaries). Others have also suggested something similar (such as Anna Freud—described in Koch, 2012; and Atkin, 1974, 1975), but the idea has not gained much traction. No doubt this is especially because this way of thinking, in terms of drives and drive transformations, is out of favour at present.

Previously in this book, and especially in the section "Repression" in chapter three, I discussed a view of repression as formed from partially neutralized aggression. These discussions built on previous arguments that I made in my book on defenses (2009, pp. 43–46), following Hartmann (1953, 1955, also Hartmann et al., 1946, 1949) for the formation of counterforce defenses such as repression, as well as other structures in the mind, from partially neutralized aggression. The formation of psychic structure from aggression is in fact often more easily observable and more "experience near," as compared to the use of libido in various functions of the mind. There is the very characteristic burst of anger that comes when a repression is challenged and that is absent when non-structural defenses such as dissociation or denial are challenged. Similarly, the aggression used to mark out a person's separation from their parents is on full display during times when the boundary between them and the parent is being built—specifically during the "terrible twos" and during the early phases of adolescence. The ability to sublimate aggression and use it for building structures in the mind is a key aspect of mental stability and resilience, including in dealing with trauma by such means as selective repression, stable identity splits, and compartmentalization.

In the case of borderline disorders I believe that the ability to sublimate libido, so that it can be stably invested in the person's self and in others, and the ability to neutralize aggression for structure building, are compromised. The issue of aggression is more obvious in the behaviour of borderlines, but I think that the problems with libido are at least as important. But what does sublimating or neutralizing libido mean? In a sense it's another way of saying what was said in the previous section about the difference between the primary process and the secondary process. In the primary process libido runs free and easy. It flits from one thing to another. Only with what Freud called its "binding" does it settle down enough to stay put for a while. This binding or neutralization tones down the intensity and easy movement of libidinal energy. It is not a question of binding being good as compared to unbound energy—each, and all the points from one extreme to another, are of use. The ability to joke or to play or to be creative in other ways requires a good dose of the flitting, unbound energy. Always sitting at the highly bound, serious end of the spectrum can create many problems. But with a general difficulty in toning down libido, borderline difficulties can ensue. As demonstrated by their ability to function at high levels at times, and sometimes for a long time, in more neutral situations such as work, borderlines, unless the disorder is very severe, are capable of drive neutralization to a reasonable extent. But in the face of stronger emotions and drives—such as family and romantic and sexual relationships—this ability reaches its limits and often breaks down. (A more severe deficit in drive neutralization is probably causative of psychotic disorders (Hartmann, 1953)).

The borderline is defined by the instability in their positive emotional investments in others, as displayed in my short example with my patient L. Another defining characteristic is what is called identity diffusion. They have the same trouble with stabilizing libidinal investment in themselves as well, and so cannot maintain a stable self image and sense of themselves. This is an emotional difficulty. They may be able to describe what they are like, but do not really feel it. As one of my patients said, "I just don't really know what I feel or want unless I have someone to bounce against—then I can be like them, or if they are too extreme from what I usually am, I can define myself by rejecting them or their ideas. When I'm by myself for too long, I turn to mush."

The unstable connection to self and others is the most obvious effect of a lack of ability to stabilize libidinal investment. In order to keep an emotionally invested image of the other in mind in their absence, one needs to tone down and modulate libido. With the deficit in this ability, the borderline is dependent on the physical presence of the other, and is often described as clinging, subject to severe abandonment anxiety, and tending to fall apart when alone for too long. The difficulty that borderlines have with synthesis, with putting different aspects of others or themselves together, and with putting even different experiences together in their mind to keep a reasonable narrative and cohesion to their lives, could be explained by the idea that the synthetic function is really a form of sublimated libido. With libido not as available for these various uses—stable investments in others, in the self, and in synthesis—more unsublimated libido is present, leading to intense sexualization of many relationships. The borderline is subject to overly strong libido not, I think, because of an intrinsically strong drive, but because of their inability to sublimate it and put it to the many uses to which it is usually put. The prominence of anger and aggression in borderline disorders can be at least partly explained in a similar manner, as a consequence of a large quantity of aggressive drive not being put to its usual uses, in building up stable repressions and stable self/other boundaries.

What has been said points to the fact that this discussion needs to take place in relation to a much more in depth consideration of development. I will again have to leave the reader with a promise that this will be provided in a book to follow, and apologize for what can only be a very superficial presentation of the issues at this point. A large amount of research has made it clear that infants are from the first related to other people, and that this does not flow secondarily from the attachment to pleasure and need for satisfaction. I would suggest that though this is true enough in that many capacities to understand, remember, and respond emotionally to others are present from very early, it is not true in relation to certain powerful emotional trends, especially aggression and libido. There is no necessary contradiction between the findings of the very early abilities in relating to others of the infant, and the ideas on drive investment being first in other things, such as the infant's own body and in feelings of satisfaction and pleasure, which then flows onto people. There is only a contradiction if we think that relating to others, and the ongoing relationship with them, is a unitary capacity born almost fully formed at an early age. Such an idea may be appealing and romantic, but it has its explanatory limitations.

It is important for the infant to be able to invest libido in, and stabilize, feelings of pleasure. Usually early unpleasureable and distressing feelings are projected outwards. With the establishment of a stable inner core of good feelings, the young child is able to tolerate the acknowledgement of some part of the unpleasant aspects of reality, thus beginning the development of what Freud (1911) called the reality principle. The borderline adult has difficulty with this. They tend to project out negative or unpleasant feelings and realities into others or into the world more generally. Thus they seem to be stuck at this early stage of the building up of the self. As Anna Freud noted (in Koch, 2012), the inability to hold onto feelings of pleasure, in essence to libidinize the self, means a child cannot make use of the mother's ministrations to build up a secure sense of themselves. This is not to say that causation of borderline problems would then be only from this constitutional factor. Observation suggests people, including young infants, vary along a spectrum in terms of this ability. An infant with moderate difficulties in this area, and a very loving, stable, and warm caretaker, would manage better than an infant with somewhat better abilities and extremely cold and/or unstable caretaking.

We can see the intolerance of unpleasant realities in the case of King Lear, who was having more than a little trouble accepting his decline and old age, and expected as a recompense that each of his daughters declare their unbounded love for him. His daughter Cordelia (perhaps an early adherent of libido theory) says that her love is limited in amount, and while she will love him as her father, she cannot declare her love for him as being infinite, as her sisters have. Lear (clearly an adherent of a different theoretical school on these matters) explodes in anger, and expels Cordelia from his kingdom. The fact that Shakespeare has Lear make this particular demand, for unbounded love, demonstrates his psychological understanding of the situation. While the borderline projects many things onto others, the one complaint that dominates is that others don't love them enough, in fact never did love them enough. And also that if only they did, things might be different. I think that this is in fact a basic primal externalization of borderlines. I believe that at some point in development, most likely around age 7 or 8, the borderline child starts to become more objectively aware that they have a problem with loving others and themselves in the way they see many others are capable of. They sense this deficit internally and project it out to others, in order to protect themselves from the intense upset and hopelessness that would come from fully acknowledging it. It is not they who are limited and hopeless, it is others. These comments are not mere speculations, as I have interpreted in this manner with borderline patients and have gotten reactions related to the awareness of this deficit, and the pain and fear it caused. (In presenting these ideas without detailed clinical material, I am aware of the limitations of this chapter, which is of necessity quite condensed, as I am trying to cover a large and complex topic in less space than it properly deserves. My excuse for doing this is that the larger project, of coming to an understanding of the deeper nature of what trauma is, and also what it is not, requires a discussion of at least some aspects of borderline disorders.)

Borderlines project out many of their internal problems, not only the inability to stabilize libidinal investment. They project out their feelings of being overwhelmed by internal forces, due to their weak repressions. They complain not only of being beset by internal feelings, but also of being traumatized by external events and things done to them. This creates a very confusing picture. And it has confused the development of theories of trauma as well, as many have taken these projections of borderlines as a starting point for theories not just about the disorder, but about trauma. We now move to tackle this confusion head on, by looking at the failure of repression in borderlines, and trying to differentiate the effects of this failure from trauma.

Repression, Internalization, and Trauma

The relationship between borderline disorders and trauma is a complex one. At its heart is a key distinction that I made early in this book, between overwhelming of the mind from outside versus from inside. Many would dispute that such a distinction even exists, and certainly many more would argue that the distinction should not be drawn too sharply. My opinion is that confusion over this issue, and the related confusion between borderline disorders and post-traumatic disorders, has obscured our view and blunted our understanding of both of these situations and their treatment.

In my book on defenses (2009) I described different sets of defenses that worked to manage impingements from outside of the mind vs such internal pressures such as drives. Affects are a kind of bridge between these two forms of impingement, as they can be powered by internal drives (sexual excitement or anxiety by libido, anger by aggression) and/or provoked by external events (sexual excitement or anxiety by a seducing person, anger by physical attack). In the section in chapter one on "overwhelming from outside versus overwhelming from inside" I outlined my theory of defenses as it pertained to this basic distinction between internal threats and external threats, as well as countering the commonly held view that equates these two. Unwanted external perceptions are usually dealt with by what I have called attentional defenses. These perceptions can be dealt with by avoidance and shifts of attention to other, more desirable realities. Attentional defenses use ego capacities such as those controlling shifts of attention (denial), thinking (intellectualization, rationalization), and differentiation (isolation) to keep distressing realities from conscious awareness. The specific internal threat of the sexual and aggressive drives exert a constant push from within the mind, and thus merely avoiding them or shifting one's attention from them is not enough, even if these are often first steps. What is usually done with such drives when they are feared (if they are not they can be simply acted on), is that an energetic counterforce is deployed to keep the drive from awareness and action.

I won't repeat myself at this point regarding the evidence that the counterforce that is the core of repression and other defenses such as reaction formation is formed from partially neutralized aggression (see Fernando, 2009, pp. 43–46, and the section "repression" in chapter two). If we assume this to be the case, however, we can gain a deeper insight not only into the dynamics of borderline disorders but also into the structure of repression. With the weakness in the capacity to neutralize the drives, we would expect that borderlines would have a weaker repression, which in fact they do. It is not that they have no ability to block dangerous or unwanted drives. For instance my patient L would often be quite unaware of the strength and content of her sexual drives, and often had a kind of general blocking of them. She could at times seem quite naive about the sexual aspects of a situation, and about her own sexual wishes. But this blocking was not the same as a stable repression. We can see this in her reaction as sadomasochistic wishes, related to past traumas, present love interests, and the transference, began to emerge in her psychoanalysis. She reacted to my interpretation with intense aggression and a projection of these wishes into me, in such a forceful manner that I felt quite destabilized. L's blocking of her sexual urges was not so stable as the selective repression of a more neurotic patient would have been. In a similar situation such a patient may also have had a burst of anger at me, but would not then explode out the whole conflict into our relationship.

An example of selective repression is presented by Peggy, who did get quite angry when I interpreted aspects of her sexual abuse. The anger did not then explode out into our relationship, but rather was defended against by reaction formations and strengthening of idealizations, as well as insight into her difficulty with the material. What made Peggy's repression of this trauma so much more secure than L's, so that it not only formed a stable structure but could then be displaced in a more differentiated neurotic transference, where she could repeat her repressed traumatic episodes and feelings? The answer I would give is that she was capable of a good deal of neutralization and sublimation of her drives, which were deployed to form a stable selective counterforce. But what does this fancy language mean?

Unneutralized aggression is like a raging child or adult who is upset or afraid of something. They may have tremendous energy to push against and defend against this thing, but it will not be very focused—they may end up destroying and lot of dishes and furniture while putting up their defense rather than selectively targeting something—and the rage will not be sustainable over time, burning out and leading to exhaustion. This is what happened in the case of L. (and also, for that matter, in the "case" of King Lear). L pushed hard against all sorts of sexual wishes, and was often surprisingly naive about the meanings of her actions.

We see something very similar to this borderline situation in the normal dynamics of early adolescence. Anna Freud (1936) described this kind of blocking leading to asceticism followed by instinctual indulgence as motivated in adolescents by a fear of the strength of the drives. Especially in early adolescence there is a normal regression and weakening of selective primal repressions as a necessary prelude to the personality being broadly and deeply restructured. Anna Freud described how the adolescent is in a precarious situation, much like the borderline. Along with this kind of non-selective and not very stable primal repression (a repression that mimics the two year old's rage reaction), we also see intense intellectual activity, including thinking about their own mental processes, as a way of binding the drive wishes. This intense intellectualism is related to the weak repressions, as secondary defenses try to do the work usually done by repression. This is something also seen in borderline patients, who are often very interested in mental dynamics and in psychoanalysis. While this can be helpful in attaching the person to therapy and the therapist, it is important to understand the deeper significance of this, rather than viewing it as a sign of "psychological mindedness," otherwise we may flood the patient by analyzing too quickly and deeply, in a situation where what the patient needs is more structure and support.

So what leads to more stable repressions? Certainly an ability to neutralize aggression helps, as the counterforce can be deployed more selectively. Peggy remembered many things about the time of the abuse, about the house, her father, and her adventures. The narrow selectivity of the repression can be seen by the fact that Peggy was able to have an enjoyable sex life with a number of partners, with the trauma showing up narrowly in her strong negative reaction if the man tried to stimulate her genitals with his hand, as her mother had done. There were other things buttressing Peggy's selective repression: she had very strong memories of the warm and friendly times with her father from childhood, and of times spent by herself on adventures. I described earlier the memory of leaving the house at a young age, walking down the busy street with trucks coming at her, and being taken in by a nice lady who gave her something to drink and had beautiful blue glass in her place (see the section "A trip down memory lane" in chapter two). This was a screen memory that contained many of the elements of the abuse, but in a reversed and denied form. There was much symbolism in the memory, including sexual symbolism, which we analyzed. This aspect of repression, the investment in screen memories, was theorized by Kris (1956b) to form part of repression. He suggested that while aggressive energy was used to block drives and memories directly, libidinal energy was invested in screen memories that buttress the repression.

The other patients whom I have presented could each be looked at from this perceptive and in each case, we could trace the dynamics of their selective repressions and the screen memories which stabilized them. For instance while Cordelia could remember the central traumatic moment of being told of her mother's death, I detailed (in the section "Repression" in chapter three) how she had repressed both the time afterwards when she felt so desperately alone, as well as her angry feelings towards her mother from before and after her illness and death, and oedipal dynamics that were tied to these. Cordelia had a general tendency to see the best in people, so as not to have her anger get carried away. I described the screen memories related to Cordelia's repression of the time after her mother's death in chapter three as well, such as the two memories involving her babysitter. I won't burden this discussion with detailed dissections of the dynamics of Cordelia, or of Joyce or Peggy, but merely say that there is enough detail in each of their case presentations for the reader to trace the dynamics of selective repression, including libidinal investment in screen memories and screen feelings.

L also buttressed her repression by investing in screens. She idealized the rather narcissistic man she had unconscious sadomasochist fantasies towards, and this played out with me as well, in an intense positive

feeling towards me and our relationship. But this was not well modulated. It quickly took on a strong sexual flavour, which made her more
scared of it. It was so intense it tended to flood out the more realistic
aspects of our relationship. And, as shown by the sequence I narrated
where this attitude towards me reversed, the repression was none too
stable. Peggy and Cordelia transferred their conflicted relationships into
the analysis, including the screening function of a positive, idealized
relationship. In its transferred form as well, the libidinal aspect of
Peggy's and Cordelia's repressions (which consisted among other things
of the investment in positive feelings and memories of their parents) was
more modulated and stable. They would joke with me and I would joke
back. There was a generally warm, friendly emotional atmosphere in the
room. What we mean by neutralization of the drive is that the aims, of
warm friendliness, were at a distance from the original sexual aims, and
the intensity was reduced, while the stability of the investments was
correspondingly increased. This leaves more room for a realistic relationship and alliance in doing the work. Not to say that more negative
and difficult feelings did not take over at times, but the more sublimated
friendly relationship was never completely blown away, and served us
well as a foundation from which to analyze these transference resistances. All of this demonstrating that the ability to neutralize libido
allowing its stable investment in a set of screen memories and screen
feelings, greatly aids in the stability of selective repressions.

These theoretical considerations related to drive neutralization and
repression may seem a bit obscure and arcane. I wouldn't suggest
bringing them up at the next party you go to, even if there are psychoanalysts present. They can be conversation killers—I can attest to that!
They are, however, quite useful in helping us understand many things
about borderline disorders, and about much else besides. In relation to
borderline disorders I believe they provide a deep explanatory framework that ties together many key features. The deficits in drive neutralization explain most easily the deficit in object constancy and the
identity diffusion, both related to not being able to stabilize investment in
one's inner representations of others or in one's own self. And the deficits
in drive neutralization lead to deficits in selective repression, and the use
instead of less selective, and less stable, blocking of drives or affects.
Because of these weak repressions, there is not as sharp a demarcation
between the primary process and the secondary process. Specifically, in
situations that involve strong feelings such as family and sexual relationships, the person becomes flooded by primary process functioning,
as described in the first section of this chapter.

Another important boundary in the mind is what Freud (1920) called the
stimulus barrier, which protects us from being overwhelmed by external
stimulation, and the breakdown of which is the beginning of trauma. Do

borderlines have a weakened stimulus barrier? And are they more prone to being traumatized? The short answer is "yes," but the more accurate answer is that it's complicated. The weakened stimulus barrier and tendency to be easily overwhelmed is only part of the problem for borderlines. Because of weak repressions and emotional instability, they are not only more prone to be beset by external impingements, but are also destabilized from the "inside" by their own drives and feelings, which are constantly getting out of control. Their barriers are weak in both directions, and this makes for a rather complicated situation, in which it is hard to distinguish the direct effects of external trauma from their interaction with poorly repressed drives and feelings and the related conflicts.

Beset from all sides, in a situation of emotional instability, and with a poor ability to distinguish fantasy from reality, or their own feelings from those of others, things are often not quite what they first appear to be in the world of the borderline. To simplify things in order to paint the big picture, I would summarize in this way: the complaints about being traumatized, which are often held up by the borderline as explanatory of almost their whole life, are projections into the external world of internal overwhelming from weak repressions. On the other hand memories of true external overwhelming leading to trauma are often avoided in much the same way by borderlines as they are by everyone else. But borderlines have difficulties compartmentalizing and metabolizing trauma to the extent done by people with better capacities to stabilize emotional investments. They tend to a much greater extent to repeat the trauma either directly or with the roles reversed. As an example if they have been abused as a child, they are more likely to get into a relationship where they are abused, or to turn around and abuse others, including their own child. In terms of the non-metabolization of trauma, I could point to Peggy's mother, who re-enacted with her a sexual abuse most likely inflicted on her by an older brother, while Peggy did no such thing with her own children, being an excellent mother, but rather had other, more internal symptoms. Peggy gained some evidence of the mother's probable abuse in visits to the uncle, her mother's older brother, as a young child. He tried forcefully to touch her genitals in the same manner that her mother had done with her. (I realize Peggy's mother was not borderline. But she demonstrates, in an even more extreme form, difficulties with internalizing and managing the zero process memories of trauma.)

It is not uncommon, in fact it is the norm, for someone with a borderline disorder to trace their difficulties to key traumas in their lives. Lear believed that all his problems stemmed from his unloving daughters. L started therapy by saying that she had had traumatic experiences in relation to a quite handsome and narcissistic man who had played with her feelings and led her on, lying about his sexual dalliances with other women. I found little reason to doubt L's description of this man. But over time, and through incidents like our interactions that I described at the start of this chapter, it became clear that her belief that what he had done to her was the cause for her problems was only part of the story, as was her belief and feeling that her father's temper and angry outbursts at L's mother and L were the cause of her difficulties with men and of her sexual difficulties. This is the sort of trauma that relates to weaknesses in repression and projection of drives. In L's case the incidents in her childhood had been upsetting and overwhelming at the time, but the strength and persistence of her reaction was striking. She was expressing a psychological truth: these incidents stood out in her mind and were connected with feelings of being overwhelmed and unable to cope. But the reason for this was her weak repressions and weakened structure more generally. L's weak stimulus barrier made what for another child would have been upsetting experiences into full blown traumas; her weak repressions meant her internal conflicts were powerfully roused by these incidents; and her weak self/other boundaries made it hard to clearly and strongly differentiate herself from her father and mother in these incidents.

The weakness of barriers and structures in many directions means that trauma, defined narrowly as overwhelming from the outside leading to zero process memories, as compared to overwhelming from inside leading to flooding and destabilization by primary process feelings and drives, are all mixed up in the case of borderlines. And they have tended to get all mixed up in our theories as well. Of course they always get all mixed up – we see this clearly enough in the dynamics I described in my patients Cordelia, Peggy, and Joyce. However, borderline disorders provide an extreme example of this mix up. Screen memories, which are a regular accompaniment of selective repression, also involve the attachment of drive conflicts onto specific external happenings, which are then often mistaken for central happenings in the person's life. A related example is the case of what are called "flashbulb memories," very distinct and strong memories for personally or socially important and often shocking events: an example being people having a strong picture of where they were and what happened when they heard of the 9/11 World Trade Centre attacks. I discussed these in the section on memory in chapter two, where I pointed out that while they sometimes enter discussions of traumatic memory, they are not zero process memories, but rather strong autobiographical memories, which are given their extra sense of importance and their intensity by the attachment of internal issues to the shocking event (for instance fears of bodily injury and conflicts over aggression can attach to a shocking attacks on the World Trade Centre). Borderlines could be pictured as living in a world full of intense flashbulb moments: incidents that hit them harder because of their weak stimulus barrier, and then intensified further as poorly repressed emotional conflicts attach to them. No wonder they feel beset by an overwhelming world.

Without the help of stable structures, borderlines suffer greatly. But they are not without tools to deal with the things that beset them. In the next section we will look at how projective identification replaces selective repression in these situations, and how it provides temporary relief, at least for the person using it.

Projective Identification, Identification with the Aggressor, and Splitting of the Identity

In my book on defenses (2009) I tried to redress the neglect of the study of repression in recent decades, and have continued these discussions at various points throughout this book, including detailing the dynamics of selective repression in this chapter. I will now present a view of projective identification as essentially what repression looks like in a situation of difficulties in drive neutralization, weak primal repressions, and compromised self/other differentiation. In such a situation, with selective repression unavailable, the individual uses projective identification as an interpersonal form of repression, used to manage drives, powerful feelings, and the zero process drives and memories left from trauma, by projecting them into another, and then mounting a severe angry boundary, the analogue of the repression barrier, between themselves and the other. In this section I will expand on these ideas and connect them to observations. I will then compare projective identification to identification with the aggressor, a maneuver with which is sometimes confused, and to the quintessential zero process counterforce defense of splitting of the identity, discussed in the last chapter.

When King Lear is told by Cordelia that her love for him is limited, his anger is volcanic. It is interesting to look at what is going on here. Cordelia has challenged a central primal denial. It is a denial held not just by narcissists and borderlines. But in more neurotic dynamics, the denial of love's limitations is buttressed by sentimental ideas and feelings, which are like the libidinal investment in screening memories and feelings that I have described as part of the structure of selective repressions. Such a selective repression and selective denial leaves room for more realistic functioning, and even intellectual knowledge of love's true nature. In Lear's case, there is no such room. He demands concrete attestations of limitless love. While his outburst at Cordelia can be seen as an indication of his narcissistic nature, I would say that at a deeper level it is an indication of, and a product of, the fragility of Lear's psyche and personality. His conflicts about love and being loved, and about aging and the decline of his powers, are not well internalized. As I described above, in terms of the lack of internalization of traumas in borderlines, the conflicts and difficulties for Lear remain external, and are acted out with his court, and especially with his daughters.

There are a number of characteristics of borderline dynamics on display here. Lear exhibits the extreme and unpredictable emotional reactivity and the lack of synthesis of object images and feelings, that I explained as a product of the intrusion of the primary process into the ego. He is to begin with extremely doting in his attitude towards Cordelia, but then there is a complete reversal. He does not merely become angry at her for not co-operating with his script of having his daughters declare their love. Rather, his entire image of Cordelia changes. From being the best of his daughters, she becomes the worst of people.

While of course we are talking about a work of fiction, what happens in the play demonstrates the dynamics of projective identification quite well. It begins with the breakdown of an already shaky defensive system, with wishes and fears and traumas threatening to flood the person. What happens next is an internal process that we largely infer from the behaviour that follows it. We can get a glimpse of it in action in the immediate aftermath of my comment to my patient L about a possible sexual meaning of her anxieties. I would see this as the analogue of Cordelia's comments to Lear—not in its content, but in its challenge to a crumbling repression. The atmosphere in the room changed immediately, and I got a very strange feeling, even though nothing was said and I could not get a good view of L's face as she was on the couch. I described it as a loud silence, and I felt very uncomfortable, even scared. I would suggest that I was feeling the effects of an internal change, in which something that L had been trying to repress—her sadomasochistic sexual wishes, and her terror of them—burst out into the interpersonal sphere. As the repression crumbles, so do self/other boundaries, and I become the carrier of these fears and drives. We could call it projection, but it is important to recognize that it is a very special type of projection, taking place in a psychological situation in which the external world and all those in it have been swallowed up into the person's mind. In this situation the repression that has crumbled internally and intrapsychically is reestablished externally and interpersonally. I contain the scary and unwanted impulses, and the interpersonal analogue of the internal repression barrier that uses partially neutralized aggression is established, also using aggression, between L and me. At this point I have disappeared as an actual person and have become, in fact have always been, a sadist intent on making L suffer.

There is much that happens in the very short span of time at the beginning of this outburst, as the intrapsychic explodes out into the interpersonal. As an observer/participant the first thing one might notice is the immediate destabilization one experiences. It happens so quickly that it can be easy to miss the depth and extent of it. One can mistake it for the mere upset or shock one might feel as someone has an angry outburst. But it is different, and this difference is key to understanding the underlying dynamics and the temporal unfolding of the process. What happens can be compared to the induction phase of hypnosis. In this, the first and very short phase, the subject's sense of reality is destabilized, leading to a regressive loss of their sense of themselves, as they become like a scared little child, in need of direction. As described in the section on dissociation in the last chapter, this allows the hypnotist to gain access to the person's mind, and some amount of authority over them. This is also what happens in projective identification. In their study of hypnosis Gill and Brenman (1961) described how subjects of hypnosis had no memory, and could not be pushed to remember, what was going on in their minds during this brief induction phase. If there was any description, they would say there was a feeling of blankness for that time. I would agree with Gill and Brenman that this lack of memory is not due to repression or some other defense, but is rather an indication of the process of regressive loss of ego functions. This process does not usually have any feelings or perceptions that would help us be aware of it. This brief period of blankness is also present just before a good joke pops into our minds – the creation of which also requires this type of regression.

The blankness and ego regression of the induction phases of hypnosis and of projective identification have some similarities with the massive ego regression that is the beginning of the traumatic process, although they do not go as deep and do not lead to a breakdown in the construction of reality and the formation of zero process memories. But they do allow access to the person's mind, either by the hypnotist or the person engaged in projective identification. One of the striking things about this access is that knowledge of what the person is doing, for instance if you are the person's therapist and have seen the projective identification play out previously, does not usually allow one to block this access. I still felt like I had to hide my sadistic personality and felt guilty after the interaction with L. Knowledge of what is going on does help one to keep the emotional reaction from spreading too far, but it enters and continues to play out for some time deep in one's emotional mind.

A better understanding of this deep and powerful emotional induction is important in comprehending abuse dynamics, and also social and political dynamics in situations with authoritarian leaders and ideologies. Let's unpack another aspect of the process—the content of the projection. I have noted that one unvarying part of the borderline's projection is the assertion that people do not love them enough, and that this lack of love is the main source of their problems. I have suggested that this core complaint and way of experiencing the world is a defensive projection of the internal perception that the person's main problem is that they themselves cannot deeply love themselves or others. Along with this basic projection, other wishes and traumas that cannot be repressed are projected into others and then the repression barrier is reestablished as an aggressive rejection of the person who now holds the difficult conflicts and traumas. As an example, we can again listen to what King Lear says to Cordelia:

By all the operation of the orbs
From whom we exist and cease to be;
Here I disclaim all my paternal care,
Propinquity and property of blood,
And as a stranger to my heart and me
Hold thee from this for ever. The barbarous Scythian,
Or he that makes his generation messes
To gorge his appetite, shall to my bosom
Be as well neighboured, pitied, and relieved,
As thou my sometime daughter.

I am not the first to note that Lear is the one who is eating up his daughters, at the very moment that he compares Cordelia to barbarians and he who eats his own children "to gorge his appetite." Lear's poorly repressed aggressive envy against the younger generation as he ages is acted out with his daughters, and when this acting out is challenged by Cordelia, he resorts to a more intense projective identification by putting his impulses into her and rejecting her and his impulses, both emotionally, as well as physically by banishing Cordelia from his kingdom.

The problem with this sort of maneuver is that it has to be resorted to repeatedly in order to maintain the person's psychological equilibrium. When this happens we often refer to the relationship as abusive. It has been stated by many authors (e.g., Novick & Novick, 1996) that there is a dynamic underlying much abusive behaviour, involving a specific way of using a person to regulate another's inner emotional life. In fact it is quite clarifying to define abuse not by actions alone, but by the presence of this interpersonal dynamic. This is especially so because the dynamic can immediately be felt by a participant or an observer. Perhaps for this reason, and also its insistent presence in the social and political landscape at the present time, this dynamic has entered into the popular imagination and become common knowledge. People will talk about being "gaslighted" by others or by political leaders, referring to the movie where a husband tries to make his wife think that she is going crazy by doing things such as putting on the light for the gas stove and insisting that she must have forgotten turning it on. There is an understanding that this kind of attempt to destabilize one's sense of reality is a first stage in getting control of one's mind. This destabilization is what I connected to the induction phase of hypnosis and the beginning phase of projective identification, involving bringing about a partial ego regression.

I have already presented a number of reasons why borderline disorders should not be considered a form of post-traumatic disorder. The dynamics of projective identification and abuse, and the interpretation of the cause and meaning of these, especially in the clinical situation, are key pieces of evidence in this argument. The way in which one feels controlled in borderline dynamics is, I would suggest, not only different from being pulled into a role in regular transferences but is also different from the counter responses of the therapist in the reenactments of trauma. That projective identification differs radically from a more structured and stable neurotic transference is obvious enough. But can we consider projective identifications as forms of intense traumatic reliving? Are they similar, for instance, to the reliving where Joyce saw me as her rapist and where I was drawn to push her as her rapist had? Joyce lost her realistic sense of who I was in the present, as did L. To repeat a short sequence from the start of chapter two: during the reliving Joyce said, "You're pulling me and pushing me now. It's not good."

"So it feels like it's now?"

"It is now. You're just pushing me too hard and I can't breathe. There's a burning in my throat. It hurts a lot."

Certainly this seems similar in its intensity and flooding of the present to L's reactions. But in many other ways it was different. I could relatively quickly become again the person in the present that Joyce knew, and we could talk about what happened. This second reality, of the rape, could at times become scarily present, but then it would recede. In the case of L and others with borderline dynamics, the distortion of reality is more ongoing. There is a general weakness in self boundaries, and in the containment of emotional life, and because of this the external world is used to manage internal conflicts. This leads to the chronic feeling of being controlled by those bearing the brunt of the projection, since in many ways they are playing a part in a play related to the other person's inner life. It would not be an exaggeration to say that the specific feeling related to borderline dynamics is the feeling that you are disappearing into the mind of the other. As the inner world of the borderline explodes out into the external world, the line between these two worlds disappears. This leads to the uncanny feelings that stay with one. I felt like a sadist not just for a moment or for a session, but long after the session with L was over. Despite the intensity of Joyce's reliving, I did not end up carrying the feeling of being her abuser. In fact the feeling that I was her abuser was not the main point of the reliving, if I can put it that way. Joyce was reliving her trauma, and as the past reality exploded into the present, I was part of the scene and was pulled into it some extent. But Joyce did not need me to be a sadistic abuser in order to rid herself of a part of herself—in fact she was perfectly happy for the whole reliving to stop and for me to go back to being my old self. Thus the invasion of the present by the past reality contained in zero process memories can be reversed rather quickly, and even when the traumatized person remains haunted by these memories, others are not. L, on the other hand, needed to keep me as the sadistic abuser.

(As a counter to this differentiation, the reader may quite rightly wonder about children who are asked to carry their parents' traumas. This topic leads very quickly into issues of development and the deposition of traumas into the superego and other places in the personality not just post-traumatically, but as part of normal human development. It is the place where the differentiation I have just made breaks down, as the zero process, the primary process, and the progressive and regressive forces of normal development come together in the transmission of ideals, fears, and many other aspects of culture, to the next generation. This will be one of the main topics of my next book. I am hopeful that the exploration of different forms of mental functioning here will facilitate new insights into their interaction in development.)

From the point of view of the outside observer and victim of their control, the borderline feels both manipulative and invasive. This leads to angry responses, and often to demonization of the individual, and of all those with borderline personality disorder. Looked at from the inside out, however, the borderline is trying to survive, to control the flooding of their mind by putting up barriers which sequester the bad impulses and bad memories in others. In a sense they are doing what we all do, they are just doing it in a different place. Usually, various memories and feelings and impulses are manipulated inside our minds—pushed away by repression into the unconscious, ignored and treated as if they did not exist through denial mechanisms, reversed into their opposites by such defenses as reaction formation, and kept sequestered one from the other by dissociative mechanisms. In the case of the borderline, these things are done with memories, feelings, and impulses now residing in the outside world, and especially in others. When L insisted that I had always been sadistic, and was angry at, and rejecting of, me, she was doing what I might have done with my own sadistic impulses, in rejecting them and setting up a strong repression barrier to keep them separate from my conscious sense of myself. The difference was that I would do it internally, while L did it with me, after she had put her sadism into me.

The weakness of mental boundaries both internally and in relation to the external world sets the stage for abusive behaviour. The flooding of the ego, and thus the relations to the external world, by characteristics of the primary process mean that the borderline is absolutely certain of their thoughts and ideas about others. Freud (1900) noted that in the primary process there is no negation. Things simply are. Negation is introduced by the growth of the ego and the secondary process. Under the influence of secondary process functioning, even a straightforward perception always has the possibility of being found to be incorrect, and thus it does not carry the same sense of absolute certainty and reality that thoughts and ideas do in the primary process. This sense of absolute certainty is contagious. It was hard to maintain my (secondary process) knowledge that I had not treated L sadistically and had not gotten sadistic pleasure from her suffering, in the face of her absolute (primary process) certainty that I had. After all, we all have some sadism—was I acting something out with her along these lines? This primary process certainty is part of the spell that the invasion of others by the borderline's mind casts over people, drawing them in. The anger that people feel around a borderline are the normal and instinctive reactions to a breaching of our boundaries, and is diagnostic of borderline dynamics. This also commonly leads to rejection and at times bullying of borderline children, and adults as well, by their peers, and by their families. Some of what a borderline reports as the uncaring, unloving treatment from their family and friends consists of these reactions. It is important in looking at the family system of a borderline not to make the same mistake that was made for so long with autistic children, and take the rejections and angry responses to the borderline as the cause of their disorder, rather than one of its effects.

Weak boundaries and the invasion of the interpersonal world by the intrapsychic and the primary process set the stage for abuse. Conceptualizing the basic borderline deficits as independent factors allows us to see not only their role in abuse dynamics but also what other factors come into play. I would say, as a generalization, that characteristics that lead to further externalization and heightened aggression are usually what lead to serious abuse, when combined with borderline deficits.

Characteristics that lead to abuse when combined with borderline deficits include narcissism, psychopathy, and traumas. In the case of narcissism and psychopathy, borderlines with these characteristics are often referred to as narcissists. While this obviously captures one part of their difficulty, it is too general. Many people with high levels of narcissism in the psychoanalytic meaning of the term—a strong libidinal investment in themselves—are not necessarily abusive. People may find them to be charming, or self-centered or, if they have stronger powers of sublimation, they may be admired as confident and accomplished. It's not just where the love is directed—whether to the self or others—that is determinative of problems, but rather what can be done with it. In the case of a borderline deficit in the ability to modulate and sublimate libido, it tends to run rampant and unmodulated. If combined with psychopathic tendencies (a deficit in empathy for others, especially for the suffering of others), serious abuse often occurs. The narcissism leads to a strong rejection of any internalization of negative observations or feelings, the psychopathic lack of feeling for others loosens any moral constraints, and the borderline tendencies towards projective identification become particularly powerful and toxic, as others are used in a manipulative and sadistic manner to manage the person's emotional difficulties. Individuals can fall victim, or whole countries.

I described previously how Peggy's psychopathic husband projected his insecurities into her. When she first met him she was confident, social, and very much engaged emotionally and intellectually in the world. He was bright, but shy and insecure. During their marriage, he consistently accused her of being incompetent and not very exciting or "with it," and also acted in ways to make her feel this way. I will give just one dramatic illustration. Peggy very much enjoyed sex. At first their sex life was good, but then her husband began more and more to use sex as a weapon and as one further way to break her spirit and self confidence. In an incident a number of years into the marriage, he had arranged for a dinner out and a nice hotel to spend the night away from the children. When she had made sexual advances in the hotel room, he rejected them angrily for reasons that she could not fathom. She gave up and went to have a bath. He then came into the washroom, dragged her out of the bath, and proceeded to rape her. Through incidents of abuse like this, and many smaller ones that wore her down, Peggy's husband made her feel both powerless and unwanted. What was striking was that even after he had managed to get most of her large inheritance when he divorced her, he still took every opportunity to use the children through what he said to them and his visits to them, to make her feel incompetent and rejected. It seemed to me that he still needed to keep projecting his sense of rejection and worthlessness into Peggy, in order to continue to feel good about himself.

Most people would call Peggy's husband, or the man who raped Joyce and then had held her hostage with the help of others, either a psychopath and/or a narcissist. This would not be wrong, but I would suggest that it would be incomplete. What would be left out would be the borderline deficit that destabilized them and led them to use projective identification and manipulation and use of the other as a way to manage this lack of structural stability. This combination of traits is dangerous in interpersonal relationships, and also in the larger social sphere. Usually in discussions on its historical and present day social manifestations as well, the narcissistic, psychopathic, and sometimes the psychotic, aspects are highlighted, while the borderline dimension is not. An exception is the study of Hitler by Bromberg and Small (1983), in which the authors detail the borderline features of Hitler's development and adult functioning, such as the splitting, impulsivity, inner emptiness, and much else. (I would say that in the study the problem was that they did not put enough stress on the other factors, which could lead to the idea every severe borderline is a potential murderous tyrant, which is not true.) The characteristics that Bromberg and Small detail are strikingly similar to a number of prominent present-day leaders, also often described or diagnosed as narcissistic. Their projection of their bad characteristics into others, whom they then demonize, is the most prominent of their borderline characteristics, but borderline dynamics are also displayed by their sudden changes of attitudes towards those around them, by their uncanny ability to set groups of people fighting one against the other (splitting), not the mention the morbid fascination with walls and keeping the demonized "other" away, a projection of their own difficulty with repression and other boundaries.

I would like briefly to turn to another defensive process that seems similar to projective identification: identification with the aggressor. Ever since the work of Ferenczi (1933), identification with the aggressor has been linked with trauma. It is always present in one way or another as an outcome of trauma, although it is certainly used more broadly than this. To get a sense of the defense, we could look at some examples given by Anna Freud in her classic book on the mechanisms of defense (1936). She described a case of August Aichhorn, the Viennese analyst who dealt with delinquent youth. A schoolboy was brought to Aichhorn because he was making strange grimacing faces in school, for which the boy had no explanation. When Aichhorn questioned the boy's schoolmaster, he noticed that the man's face when he got angry talking about the boy's behaviour bore a resemblance to the boy's grimaces. Aichhorn surmised that the boy was actually quite scared of the schoolmaster, and that when he became anxious that the man would punish him, he identified with his angry face through his grimaces. Thus, at the level of fantasy and action, he exchanged the position of terrified schoolboy for a terrifying schoolmaster, providing temporary protection against his fears.

In this somewhat older boy, the mechanism was unconscious. Anna Freud also described an example of the conscious use of this device in a younger patient of hers who was scared of seeing ghosts in the hallway of her house. She would run across the hallway gesticulating wildly. She explained to her brother that as long as you pretend to be the ghost you might meet you were safe. In this explanation the little girl captures perfectly the basic mechanism of identification with the aggressor. Often, however, this simple maneuver is supplemented by others, most commonly turning passive into active and projection of aspects of the self into others. Another of Anna Freud's young patients demonstrated this combination of defenses. As wishes and fantasies related to masturbation threatened to emerge in his therapy, he became quite aggressive. He tried to hit his mother and nurse and eventually took knives from the kitchen and threatened them with these. Analysis of these actions showed that the little boy was afraid of physical punishments and castration from the very people he attacked, related to his masturbation. Here he identified with his potential attackers but also turned the tables on them, making them the frightened and vulnerable ones, not himself.

As Anna Freud's examples make clear, identification with the aggressor is a common way that children deal with scary or upsetting attacks, whether traumatic or not, and whether these attacks have already occurred or are merely feared. The "aggressor" with whom the person identifies may not attack. There can be identification with the neglector, a very common maneuver in which the child neglects or rejects others rather than being the abandoned one. The basic maneuver of identification with the aggressor involves switching places with another in order to defend against distressing feelings. One can also identify with an attacking introject or superego, where one spares oneself the distress of being attacked by these introjects by attacking others as one would otherwise be attacked.

But what about the relation between identification with the aggressor and projective identification? Are they perhaps just versions of the same thing? While they both have the word "identification" in their name, identification with the aggressor involves selective identification with certain characteristics of the attacker or depriver, used as a defense, while projective identification involves projection of an unwanted drive, memory, etc. into another, in the context of weak self/other boundaries. The term "identification" in projective identification is used because the person is thought to still keep a connection or identification with the part of them that they have projected. For instance, L still felt identified with the sadism that she accused me of, which was the reason she needed to induce it in me and reject it so strongly. This identification is an effect of the weak self/other boundaries, which leads to the internal world exploding out into the external one. So, to the extent that I was in a sense swallowed up into L's mind, of course what she imputed to me also belonged to her. But it is only in this very special sense that projective identification involves identification—a very different type of identification than identification with the aggressor.

These two different types of identification in these two defenses are a product of their very different natures. When Anna Freud's little patient waves her arms wildly to pretend to be a ghost, this is selective identification, related to the functioning of the organized secondary process. Identification with the aggressor is a defense that uses attentional and other abilities of the ego to defend against unpleasant realities, such as a ghost or a scary schoolmaster. It is a secondary process attentional defense. By contrast, L dealt with her crumbling repressions by projecting her sadism into me, and then using an aggressive counterforce to separate herself from me and from her sadism that now resided in me. Projective identification is an interpersonal counterforce defense that uses the nature of the primary process as well as intense aggressive rejection (the "counterforce") to aid in projecting a drive into another person and making sure that it stays there. The analyst becomes highly embroiled in the patient's dynamics in this defense. The process informs us about the structural state of the person's ego (weak repressions) and about the drive conflicts that are insecurely repressed. Identification with the aggressor is a denial defense deployed against overwhelming unpleasant real experiences and internal realities such as an attacking superego. The defense does not embroil the analyst to as great an extent and is for this and other reasons often difficult to spot and analyze – despite its ubiquity and importance. The defensive process and its analysis inform us about important, overwhelmingly distressing reality or fantasied situations, whether internal or external, past or present.

Identification with the aggressor is a ubiquitous dynamic, both in relation to trauma and in non-traumatic situations. It hides in plain sight, and is often missed. At times it comes to the attention of others, such as a schoolboy who makes strange faces, but it does not intrude on others in the manner of projective identification. Peggy kept trying to tidy her place up and get rid of clutter. Once she had done that, she said, she could finally get to the things she wanted to do, like write and paint. But this never happened. The connection with various dynamics, including the sexual abuse by her mother and a repetition of being in the mess and disorder of her mother's house and her mother's mind as a child were analyzed, with little change. I then interpreted that perhaps she was being like her mother in not being able to declutter her place. In doing this she protected herself from being the little girl who was overwhelmed by a chaotic place, a mother's chaotic mind, and the smell and feel of the sexual abuse. She was instead the oblivious mother who embodied the chaos and dirt. I can't say Peggy liked this interpretation, but it led to strong feelings and movement in relation to the feelings of mess in the present, which had not happened with any of the other interventions.

Peggy's reactions and resistances were typical of those for an attentional defense. She did not like the interpretation, but there was not the burst of anger that you see with counterforce defenses. Rather, she got confused when trying to understand it, went back to just talking about the repetition without the identification, then would change the topic, and then finally forgot that I had ever mentioned it. This is typical with denial as well—often an intellectual agreement, but then a slippery loss of the insight. I have a feeling that this slippery loss of an important insight has happened within psychoanalysis as a whole as well in relation to identification with the aggressor, which is not explored and interpreted as much as its frequent centrality in post-traumatic and other dynamics would dictate.

And what of splitting of the identity in contrast to projective identification? Here the two defenses are unlikely to be confused with each other, but they do make for an interesting and enlightening comparison. I have already described (in the last section of chapter three) splitting of the identity as a compound defense involving dissociation and counterforce between identities containing different aspects of a trauma. To put it in simpler terms, splitting of the identity is what repression looks like in the zero process. Using the same formula, we could say that projective identification is what repression looks like in the primary process.

With these formulas in hand, we might be led to a number of further questions. If splitting of the identity is a compound defense, which I think all clinical evidence of the nature of the resistance faced when analyzing it argues that it is, then is projective identification also a compound defense? Does it involve a counterforce acting in concert with other aspects of the primary process, such as easy displacement, lack of negation, and porous self other boundaries? The short answer I would give is "yes," although a proper theoretical description of the situation would necessitate further explication of the nature of compound defenses, which is beyond the scope not only of this chapter but of this book, and is something I will undertake in my next book, in concert with an exploration of the nature of obsessionality, of the building up of the internal object world, and of the development of the superego.

But one thing we can answer in more detail here are the clinical implications of our theoretical explication of the dynamics of these defenses. How do we approach these dynamics, and more generally the zero process as compared to the primary process? Do we need additions or modifications to the techniques developed first to analyze primary process/secondary process dynamics, and more recent changes proposed to analyze early development and the growth of the self? This is the central question of the next chapter.

Chapter 5

Therapeutic Technique in Analyzing Post-Traumatic States

Approaching the Zero Process

Early on in the exploration of trauma, Pierre Janet realized that in trauma, the present moment had come to a halt, and he suggested therapeutic strategies of getting patients to finish actions that had been halted by the trauma. He used hypnosis both to suggest that things were different, and more positive, than the actual trauma that had happened, and also to take the person back into the trauma so that they could finish processing it, and have it finally put to rest as a memory of the past. Janet also suggested reversing the feelings of being overwhelmed and of defeat during the trauma by taking the person back into the trauma and having them then play out a different response than actually occurred (Van der Hart & Friedman, 2019). Many modern techniques are related to, and sometimes explicitly derived from, Janet's work.

As an example, sensorimotor therapy works in a "bottom up" manner, starting from physiological and action responses of the body, and attempting to finish actions halted by the trauma, or to fashion new actions that did not occur at the time. To give a flavour of this work, I quote from the book by Pat Ogden (the originator of this therapy) and her collaborators: "[a]s clients begin to explore these defensive tendencies in a mindful way, a spontaneous phenomenon often occurs: the mobilizing defensive responses begin to present themselves in the body: a tightening of the jaw, arms, and fist or sensations in the throat accompanied by a feeling of wanting to speak or scream. Through the slow and painstaking work of observing what the body wants to do as the trauma is recalled, the possibility of a new response emerges, incipient during the original trauma, ready to be further developed into defensive responses that are more flexibly adapted to the present" (Ogden et al., 2006, p. 107). They conceptualize this as working at the sensorimotor (reptilian brain) level, because some of the responses at this level become fixated and stuck at the time of the trauma. They contrast this with the affective, old mammalian

DOI: 10.4324/9781003283218-6

(paleo-mammalian, limbic system) part of the brain, and the cognitive, or neo-mammalian and cortical, level.

Many other therapies use non-verbal modalities to get at traumatic memories. These include art therapy, various movement therapies including dance/movement therapy (Sandberg & Tortora, 2019), drama therapy, and different types of massage therapies that attempt to unlock memories that are held in muscle tensions. In his popular book on trauma, Van Der Kolk (2014) describes Eye Movement Desensitization and Reprocessing (EMDR), yoga, internal family systems therapy (where part of the person and their defenses are objectified as separate entities), psychomotor therapy (a specific technique using props for people in the patient's life), and neurofeedback. Each of these techniques aims to get at dissociated memories that have not been given verbal labels or been linked to the regular narrative memory networks of the individual. Using our terminology, we could see them as attempting to access zero process memories through using modalities that connect with the nature of these memories. More specifically, because the memories are concrete, lack abstraction, lack language, and are in bits and pieces, with different sensory modalities such as a smell or a sound or a pull to action not connected with each other, these techniques start with little pieces of the concrete and the non-verbal: with a tight jaw, or a tendency to lift one's arm to protect oneself. They also, similar to the zero process, concretize experiences, such as having a piece of furniture stand for a person in psychomotor therapy, or the personification of parts of the mind in internal family systems therapy. Some, such as EMDR and neurofeedback, are specifically targeted at the overstimulation and hyperarousal connected with traumatic reliving; allowing the person to access and process the trauma without being overwhelmed. To the extent that they are used for trauma work, these techniques attempt to access zero process memories from the trauma directly, on their own terms and at their own level, rather than attempting to reach down to them from above, with language and conceptual thought.

Along with techniques that directly mirror the concrete nature of the zero process, hypnosis and suggestive techniques were also first championed by early investigators such as Janet. These mirror not just the nature of zero process memories, but also the process of their formation through the regressive loss of ego functions during trauma. In hypnosis this regression is controlled and put to use. I described aspects of hypnosis and hypnotic induction in the section on dissociation in chapter three, and in the last chapter when describing projective identification. Hypnosis is a special type of controlled regression, where some ego functions are suspended for specific purposes. The hypnotist replaces the person's superego, or inner parent, as the person regresses to the position of a dependent child who is told what is real and what to do by the hypnotist/parent.

Trauma is too much happening too fast. What we want to achieve in order to analyze trauma is to have smaller bits happen more slowly. Hypnosis and similar techniques, used in conjunction with other methods, or separately, have this general aim. In the case of the aftereffects of truly horrendous and overwhelming trauma, leading to dissociative identity disorder, Kluft (2013) maintains that hypnosis used by a therapist well trained in the technique is an absolute necessity, in order to control the appearance and behaviour of various alters and protect the patient from the sometimes dangerous acting out of some alters. Hypnosis is used to bring order to an overwhelming and chaotic situation of many alters, each formed around specific sets of zero process memories (see the section on dissociative identity disorder in chapter three), taking control of the person's conscious awareness and actions. Kluft (1997, 2013) describes a "fractionated abreaction" technique, where smaller bits of the trauma are allowed to play out, with hypnosis and/or other techniques used to stop the reliving after it has only gone a small way. Others (e.g., Maldonado & Spiegel, 1998) also describe various techniques, which can involve, as an example, picturing a screen on which the traumatic memories are projected as they emerge, keeping them at some distance, but also giving the person control of them. They could then picture that they are able to turn off the video, freeze it, make it go more slowly so that they can comprehend it, etc. Another common technique is to picture a safe place, absolutely soothing and comforting, to which the patient can go during the trauma work.

Similarly to somatic and non-verbal therapies, these hypnotic techniques attempt to meet the post-traumatic memories where they reside—in the world of present realities. They include not just the hypnosis, but the instructions given using hypnosis, such as that an alter should go to sleep, and such techniques as the use of projection of the memories onto a screen. And there is the way in which alters are treated and talked to as if they were different people, not just as aspects of the person, or as fantasies. This type of work can seem either mystical or naive to psychoanalysts, many of whom would see the alters as memory/fantasy complexes forming internal objects. However, to the extent that alters are zero process structures, they exist as entities in the present, something quite different from a fantasy or a regular memory of the past. Treating them as a fantasy or an animated set of memories from the past would in many cases be a technical mistake. Such an attitude would not address the zero process nature of the alters and other memories and symptoms. Kluft (2013) notes that treating alters as realities is actually a key to undoing their independent existence and reintegrating them into the self system. We have to approach the zero process on its own terms, in order to bring the memories it contains back into the fold of our regular self and regular way of being in the world. What Kluft says about alters in

DID applies more generally to zero process symptoms and structures. It is necessary to treat them as realities if one is to turn them into past memories, and reintegrate them.

Having made these observations about approaching the zero process on its own terms, what are we to make of the psychoanalytic talk therapy for traumatized patients such as I have described in this book, and used as a basis for building up the theory of the zero process, and for illustrating it? Not only does the psychoanalytic method allow a deep and wide ranging view of the mind, but it allows us also to test various hypotheses we may develop. It has been enormously helpful to me and others in developing our ideas and building our models of trauma. But let's look now at its uses, and problematics, in dealing with trauma clinically. The light regression fostered by lying down, the frequency of sessions, and asking the patient to relax their self criticisms and say whatever comes to mind, allows the interplay of forces within the patient's mind to come to light. It also over time fosters certain types of transferences: displacements of early relationship patterns, and of powerful drive wishes and feelings onto the therapist and the therapy situation. Freud (1913a) stated that the therapist "sets in motion a process, that of the resolving of existing repressions. He can supervise this process, further it, remove obstacles in its way, and he can undoubtedly vitiate much of it. But on the whole, once begun, it goes its own way and does not allow either the direction it takes or the order in which it picks up its points to be prescribed for it" (p. 130).

What drives this process, in the classical conception, is, literally, the drives: the sexual and aggressive drives pushing for expression, that are helped along by the relaxation of the defenses and their interpretation. Their push for expression displaces into the analysis, and so we get the transferences. While the psychoanalytic process does have, as Freud noted, a surprising degree of independence from the efforts of the analyst, that does not mean that the analysis runs itself. For one thing, the analyst has to set the process in motion, by setting the frame of the treatment and connecting with the patient enough that they attach to the analyst and the analysis. And when things come to a head, with powerful transference reliving and transference resistances, the analyst has to manage them, make sense of them, and interpret them by tracing them to their origins. Still, while the analysis does not run itself, it has a certain momentum and direction all its own.

The reader may object that this is an old-fashioned model of analysis, that doesn't take into account modern innovations. I will get to this in a moment, but will first use this simple scheme to ask, how does trauma fit into the psychoanalytic process? One problem is that zero process memories are by their very nature dissociated from the large mass of more regular memories and from regular functioning. This is one reason that techniques such as sensorimotor therapy, drama therapy, and others mentioned at the start of this section were developed—to allow access to zero process memories by engaging with them at their own level and in their own form. A second problem is that once engaged traumatic memories can repeat in a manner that is too overwhelming—this is usually the reason that they were dissociated, repressed, or otherwise defended against in the first place. Many techniques not only help with access but with modulation of the reliving, while other supplementary interventions, such as EMDR, and certain drugs such as MDMA, are also used to help with modulation.

The first problem, of the dissociation of the traumatic memories, means that they cannot be expected to reliably show themselves in a regular analysis or therapy by virtue of the analytic process alone. Of course emotional conflicts also will not declare themselves openly but various derivatives, including those in the transference, can be expected to show up, and be amenable to being worked with, as the therapy moves along. Not so with zero process memories. They will show up unreliably, when they are triggered by specific and impossible to predict external or internal events. One will notice them by the presence of specific reactions that seem strangely out of character and to come from nowhere. Not to say that one cannot access traumas through regular dynamic therapies or psychoanalysis, but the basic set up can work against this, if one is not flexible and does not take into account the special nature of post-traumatic reactions, and is not on the lookout for zero process memories.

In terms of recent advances in psychoanalytic technique, while they have allowed us to better analyze certain issues, I believe that they can also work against recognizing trauma and treating it. This may seem a surprising thing to assert, given the extent to which trauma has been talked about and theorized about in recent literature, but there are a number of reasons for this. Firstly, the concentration on gaining access to the patient's mind through one's countertransference, and on the therapy being a product of the transference/countertransference interactions and developments, can work against recognizing zero process memories, which only unpredictably and unreliably enter into the transference/countertransference matrix. Secondly, the decline of interest in, and at times active hostility towards, reconstructing what happened in the patient's past (with the exception of very early mother/child interactions), works against our ability to analyze these zero process memories in a way that is therapeutically helpful, once we have recognized them. And thirdly, the newer relational ideas, while leading to helpful innovations and advances in techniques, have over time (at least in some quarters) become quite reductive, with development, symptomatology, and therapy all reduced to two person interactions and mutual creations, and trauma has been caught up in this reduction, being redefined as what one person does to another, usually during very early childhood; leaving many other forms of trauma, many other determinants, and many other ages when trauma can occur, out of the picture.

The difficulties that trauma presents to psychoanalytic therapy can be divided into those brought on by a too rigid and reductive technique, such as looking always for drive conflicts, or insisting on analyzing only within the transference/countertransference matrix, and those difficulties related to more basic aspects of psychoanalysis, such as reliance on language and being relatively non-directive. These core aspects are not only difficulties but also of course strengths of psychoanalysis. By using free association and evenly hovering and wide ranging attention on the part of the analyst, many of the connections traumatic memories have made with other issues can be explored. As an example, we could think of the links made by Cordelia between death and aggression, so fatefully tied together early in her life. We discovered not only her anger at her mother for leaving through death, but its connection with earlier rage at the birth of her siblings, and oedipal aggression and wish to get rid of her mother that was starting to bubble up as her mother got ill and then died. Cordelia's difficulty in using her aggression productively, as well as her difficulties in romantic relationships, were traced to these connections, and also to a central happening when she was in early adolescence, when her father married her stepmother. This brought on a host of feelings, including hope for a mothering relationship, unconsciously connected to a fantasy that her mother had returned, as well as anger and oedipal sexual jealousy in relation to the marriage. Her stepmother proved harsh and punitive, interfering with Cordelia's attempts during adolescence to rework her oedipal issues, conflicts over aggression, and earlier traumas. These interferences came to a head in Cordelia's early adulthood, leading to physical symptoms and difficulties in relationships that she did not know the origins of.

Despite the uncovering of all these connections, in Cordelia's case, and in all cases of trauma, the unconstructed zero process memories act as anchors, holding down and not allowing the working through of all the conflicts and happenings to which they become connected. Thus one may uncover and analyze all sorts of dynamics and yet see little change. As one example to stand for the rest I will mention again the case of a five-year old boy presented by Alvin Frank (1969) that I described in the first section of chapter two ("Traumatic Memories and the Construction of Reality"). The boy had a powerful wish to be tied up, which pushed aside all other interests. Frank had worked with him for a while in psychoanalysis, but it was only when the trauma of his mother having tied him up all day in a high chair for a month long period when he was eight months old had come to light, and she had described it to her son, that the wish to be tied up lost its intense and obsessive hold on him. There was still work to be done in the analysis, Frank noted, but after this, many other conflicts and issues which had stubbornly persisted, despite diligent efforts, yielded to therapeutic work.

It is its ability to not just analyze traumas, drive conflicts, developmental interferences, and much else but, most crucially, the ability to analyze the interactions of all these factors, that is the strength of psychoanalytic therapy. But in order to be able to take advantage of these in relation to trauma, psychoanalytic therapy needs to be able to approach the zero process. This certainly happens all the time in dynamic therapies. But it also happens all the time that traumas are missed or downplayed or confused with other phenomena or not pursued in enough depth. There can be any number of reasons for these difficulties but I would like, in the rest of this chapter, to explore how specifically our study of the zero process can help us to understand how trauma appears in therapy, to recognize it, and to analyze it. In the previous chapter, we compared zero process manifestations with those primary process and developmental manifestations exemplified especially in borderline disorders. In the next section, we will look at the therapeutic implications of these differentiations. In chapter two and especially chapter three, I introduced ideas about post-traumatic dynamics related to the zero process drive and zero process defenses. In the last section of this chapter I will further elaborate these ideas and present specific interventions that are helpful in the analysis of trauma dynamics. But before embarking on these explorations, it may be worthwhile to consider the most basic of defenses related to trauma, and the importance of reconstruction of the traumatic reality based on information from outside the therapy.

Kluft (2000) notes that in DID patients an important defense is reluctance: "[o]ften, repression, dissociation, resistance, and reluctance are all operative in a particular clinical incident, but it is the clinical approach to reluctance, often based on shame, threats of punishment for sharing the information, or some conflict in the inner world of the personalities, that characterizes the successful resolution of DID psychopathology" (p. 262). While reluctance and avoidance may be especially strong in DID, they are important reactions in every trauma therapy. This makes sense in terms of the theory of the zero process: because the zero process memories behave as present experiences, the person naturally reacts to them as they would to any extremely distressing or threatening present experiences—they attempt to escape them. In keeping with the immediate nature of these zero process memories, the escapes are often strongly physical. Peggy put her hands over her face as we talked about her psychotic mother. "I can see her eyes and it makes me shiver," she said. "My whole body is so tight and tense. I didn't realize how tense I was last session when we talked about her until after the session."

In the face of this reluctance and avoidance, a judicious amount of active confrontation is helpful. This can involve merely pointing out the avoidance—something like, "you really drop that topic whenever we come close to it." I said this to Peggy, and I also commented on her covering her face and how hard it was for her to look at her mother and at the situations with her. I would at times push for a bit against the avoidance, along with asking for associations and making interpretations about what I thought it might be specifically related to. Confrontation doesn't mean sticking to the ideas you have about a trauma no matter what the patient says. It means bringing up the memories that are avoided and pointing out the persistent avoidance, and then giving the patient time and space to internalize what you have said, to respond, to associate, and then being guided by their responses. It means bringing up the topic of a trauma with overwhelming feelings early in the session, so that the upset can be worked on, and then helping to wind down the exploration in the last third of the session. It means being flexible enough to spend time on the analysis of emotional conflicts, transference manifestations, and developmental influences such as deprivations and over-gratifications, as they emerge through the patient's associations, rather than getting caught up in pursuing avoided traumatic memories no matter what.

This last point requires subtle judgements. At times when one pushes against the patient's avoidance of traumatic memories, changing the topic and concentrating on other issues will be much in evidence and quite transparently defensive. At these times, I think it is worth pointing this out and persisting with the pursuit of the zero process memories. At other times, associations will lead to things connected to the traumatic memories, and it will be helpful to spend time on these. Each of the more extended clinical vignettes from Cordelia, Peggy, and Joyce demonstrate both the interpretation of avoidance, and the emergence of other connections that were not simply avoidance, and that deepened our analysis of the trauma. A rather extreme example of active confrontation of avoidance was in evidence in the sessions where memories of her violent rape emerged in Joyce's analysis that I detailed at the start of chapter two, in introducing the idea of the zero process. I will discuss this example of active confrontation further in the next section.

Reluctance and avoidance are not something displayed only by patients. There is a specific counter resistance exhibited by the therapist in relation to trauma. In the section on memory in chapter two I described a study by Gaensbauer and Jordan (2009) in which they interviewed therapists about childhood trauma, and when they reinterviewed the therapists many had forgotten about the traumas from their own patients that they had talked to the researchers about on the first occasions. Of course counter reactions to the traumas of our patients are varied and complex, and include also overemphasizing traumas and reducing all of a patients problems to one or a few traumas. In fact these two reactions belong in the same category, of therapists mirroring both trauma avoidances and trauma screening of patients. They are ubiquitous and unavoidable, and if the therapist becomes adept at spotting them in themselves, they can also be invaluable guides. Let me give just one example.

I have already described, in the section "Repression" in chapter three, how Cordelia's memory of her father telling her about her mother's death was not just a trauma in its own right, but its strong remembrance screened the repressed time of emptiness and desolation in the months after. We were led to this time by noticing the gap in memory, and slowly the memories and feelings emerged from repression. Another memory was mentioned by Cordelia a number of times during her therapy, including at the start. She had spent time in hospital at around the age of three, after she came down with croup. She remembered clawing her way out of the netting over her crib, and wandering the halls of the hospital. Neither she nor I lingered very long over this memory. I remember having a passing thought that this was not so important, and being vaguely annoyed that it was a distraction from the work at hand. I was somewhat more enthusiastic about references in dreams and Cordelia's associations, to her pained reaction to the birth of her siblings. Here I was more drawn to analyzing her reactions to her sister's birth, when she was three, than her brother's birth when she was 11 months old. "You can't remember much from that age, can you?" asked Cordelia, when this birth came up.

To make a very long story very short, much further along in Cordelia's therapy, later than any of the sessions described in this book, the analysis of these two incidents allowed us to understand much more deeply her terror of abandonment, and her feelings of anger, jealousy and being left out. These feelings had kept appearing in dreams and her feelings and actions in her present life, and had been analyzed both in relation to other traumas and various emotional conflicts. However, it was only once I realized my counter resistance, in downplaying the two early traumas, and we had gone into the details, that there was deeper movement in Cordelia's fears and feelings of jealously and being left out. This is another demonstration of the manner in which core zero process memories anchor all sorts of other dynamics and traumas, which only prove analyzable and moveable once the anchor is loosened. The horror as she was left alone for the night in the hospital by her visiting father, which mounted as she clawed at the netting over her crib, were intensely lived out by Cordelia in therapy. She also recovered memories—mainly emotional memories and some vague perceptual ones—related to the shock of seeing her mother stroke and pet her newly arrived brother when she was 11 months old.

My more specific purpose in touching on the analyses of these early traumas is that they demonstrate the operation of my counter reaction of dismissal and avoidance. It was only once I spotted this resistance on my part that I was freed up to help Cordelia by taking her associations related to these traumas seriously. Each therapist needs to become conversant with the form trauma avoidance and minimization takes for them. The more general aspects are that the thought that the association may be important is felt but said in a soft voice, which is easily dismissed. As a general rule, if one is tempted to dismiss such associations—an analogue of the patient's avoidance of trauma—they are much more likely to be valid than when one feels very insistent on one's ideas.

These examples are also a good opportunity to put in a word for the importance of constructing the traumatic past. In all the instances of analysis presented in this book, reconstructions of buried forgotten times was important. In the case of Joyce, we gained access to her repressed period of captivity especially by talking to an alter, a young adult Joyce, and working on the hatred this alter and a care taking alter had for each other, which worked against the awareness and integration of memories that they each held. While my own countertransference played a part in the analysis of this time, it was not centre stage. We were reconstructing a whole piece of Joyce's forgotten history, and only some parts of it played out with me. Even for many of the parts that did, they only started playing out once we had done a lot of detective work, involving talking to the alter, looking at Joyce's symptoms, reliving of physical responses inside and also out of the analysis, defense analysis, and much else.

The building up of the narrative, and the importance of its accuracy, should not be underestimated in its power to spur the emergence of repressed and dissociated traumas. It can set a virtuous circle going, in which as the zero process memories from traumas emerge and are put into the past, they enrich the narrative further, leading to the emergence of more memories. Some warn of the dangers of this sort of work in that you can start to construct false memories, and sometimes this worry is used as an argument to approach the past only through the transference. I would argue that the transference is prone to the very same sources of error as work outside of the transference. If you take a naive view of either source of evidence, believing that one's feelings and thoughts during the therapy give one privileged access to the patient's past, or believing that one should always believe the patient in whatever they assert about their trauma, one can be led to construct false narratives and false memories. But the best protection against these dangers is an open minded and flexible technique that follows the patient's associations where they lead, rather than where you or the patient think they should lead, as well as an understanding of the nature of memory, of mental dynamics, of screen memories, and of the different forms of mental functioning.

The disinclination to make assertions about external reality works in tandem with the patient's own avoidance and denial as well as, in the case of those who have been physically, sexually, or psychologically abused, mirroring the abuser's gaslighting of the patient and attempts to destroy their ability to know what actually happened. One will be pulled into this kind of denial no matter what, as part of the normal resonance with the patient's denial, but it is not helpful if the therapist also has theoretical and clinical ideas that push them further in this direction. The point is not to replace denial and gaslighting with false certainty, but to replace it with a mature and rational attitude towards reality. With this attitude, one can pay attention in an even-handed manner to the various realities of the patient's past, and construct with the patient a reasonable narrative of what happened to them.

Present day reactions outside of the therapy and transference are often important sources of information. Anniversary reactions are ubiquitous. Also common are the triggering of traumas by children. Generally, specific traumas will be triggered as the child of a person reaches the age when the trauma took place. In people with a lowered ability to internalize and repress traumas, they may be acted out with the child. I have mentioned how Peggy's mother sexually abused her, almost certainly in the manner, and perhaps at the age, when the mother was sexually abused by her older brother. I have seen patients who were beaten by a parent when they reached the same age that the parent was beaten. In many instances, the acting out of the trauma will be toned down in its severity. It is a good general rule that one should keep an eye out for the interactions, and the possibility that you are not being told about abusive interactions, between patients and their children. In many instances, patients will try to steer towards their own abuse as children, avoiding the guilt and shame brought about by what they are doing to their own children, by talking about themselves as victims. But these interactions with their children are the living, beating heart of their past trauma, with their own fear and other feelings, now acted out projected onto their own children, and their own avoidance of realistic guilt mirroring their parent's avoidance.

Anniversary reactions and reactions with children are merely some of the more common repetitions triggered by situations with concrete similarities to aspects of the trauma. Many of the reactions related to children, especially in patients with better psychic structure and better ability to repress and sublimate, do not involve repeating the abuse they have suffered, and yet are informative and worth analyzing. I described how Peggy was an excellent mother who created an atmosphere at home with her children quite the opposite of what she had experienced with her mother. The connection with the past was revealed by the fact that when she could not do this any more, because of the divorce and her ex-husband's use of the children against her, the loneliness and terrible feeling of being unloved by her mother flooded back into her life.

Creating a loving and playful family life in a beautiful home was a sublimatory reversal of Peggy's experience with her own mother, and it kept the zero process memories at bay.

Patients will also develop symptoms based on their child's age. A patient finally came to see me after many years of her physical symptoms being misdiagnosed as neurological. They turned out to be related to sexual abuse by an uncle who had slept in the same room as her. The abuse had started when she was two, and during the therapy it emerged that her very debilitating physical symptoms had started when her daughter reached two. This patient also was a very good mother, demonstrating the neurotic solution to traumatization involving repression, in her case splitting of the identity, and generally internalizing reactions, versus externalization the abuse. Analysis led to a quick diminution of her symptoms. We did good work for a number of years, on the splitting of identity, and on striking physical symptoms. Then there was a sudden, almost complete, loss of many of her symptoms, which was gratifying and a bit surprising. I wondered about a transference meaning, or perhaps the effects of my brilliant interpretations. But no, it turned out that her daughter had reached the age when the abuse had stopped. A couple of years later, there was a sudden eruption of symptoms that was short lived. Her daughter had reached the age when her uncle had cornered her and raped her, one last time.

At this point in the discussion, having outlined the relationship of the concept of the zero process to some basic concerns in trauma therapy, it is time to compare these to work with borderline disorders and serious developmental interferences. Just as exploring more deeply the characteristics of the primary process allowed us to bring the nature of the zero process into focus, and elucidating borderline dynamics based on the invasion of the ego by the primary process allowed us a deeper insight into the contrasting invasion of ego by the zero process in posttraumatic disorders, so will an excursion into the therapy of borderline disorders and developmental disorders allow us to bring into focus the nature of trauma therapy. Thus, we will consider this topic before we conclude with a discussion of the analysis of zero process dynamics.

The Relation of the Analysis of the Zero Process to Analysis of Other Phenomena

While the rediscovery of older works on trauma, and interest in such authors as Janet (1920) and Ferenczi (1933) has led to important new therapeutic ideas and advances, the confusion that began over a century ago between post-traumatic phenomena and other manifestations remains, both in those who follow Janet and within the psychoanalytic literature. I have pointed out that the idea of a different form of mental functioning after trauma is not so original—in fact it is quite old. What is more original in zero process theory is the attempt to look more deeply into these phenomena, and by so doing to differentiate post-traumatic mental functioning from the functioning in the deeper unconscious (the primary process), to disentangle these both from effects of developmental interferences, and to differentiate different forms of dynamics in the same person. I discussed this whole issue at length in the last chapter, as well as in chapter two when I introduced the idea of the zero process. I don't propose at this time to go into detail about the treatment of borderline disorders or of developmental disorders—a very large and complex topic indeed. Rather, my aim is to identify the ways in which the confusion I have been exploring impacts on the treatment of trauma, and to make some comments that may be helpful in disentangling the clinical presentation and the treatment of different dynamics.

A good place to start may be the point I have made about the importance of being active, and working against the patient's avoidance, in seeking out traumas. There are a number of reasons for resistance to this idea. In many case presentations to audiences and cases in the literature, the therapist takes the stand that the patient is not ready yet for deeper exploration of a trauma, and that much work has to be done before they will be ready. Of course active confrontation of avoidance has to be done judiciously, judging when the patient is stable enough and feeling safe enough. But if one follows the patient's feelings on the matter, at some point as one evokes zero process memories, they will feel that it is not a good time and that they are not ready. In fact, in terms of these feelings, there is never a good time to live out the trauma. This attitude on the part of someone who has been traumatized is the norm. It is a reliving, in fact a zero process memory, of the experience of going into a situation in the actual trauma for which they were not prepared.

What to do in such a situation? Many of the hypnotic and quasi-hypnotic techniques that have been developed, such as tapping and EMDR, are ways of circumventing or calming down these overwhelming feelings. Also, with truly overwhelming and complex traumas, with full blown DID, hypnosis or other techniques are necessary (see as an example the case of Ira Brenner's (2004) in which he introduced EMDR). Some of the experiments with using drugs in relation to exploring trauma also attempt to do this, for instance in the use of MDMA and psychedelics such as LSD. This is a quickly developing field. But at this point I would like to address the problem directly from within a standard psychotherapy framework. I believe this is one among many areas where not distinguishing clearly between borderline disorders, other ego deficits, and the zero process is detrimental. In the case of borderline disorders there is often an uncontrolled regression as one opens up serious traumatic incidents, which does not resolve easily, and which is not therapeutically helpful. What is necessary in handling these situations should not be overgeneralized to the handling of trauma in those with more resilient structures and better ego capacities.

In order to bring the clinical aspects into focus, let's circle back to the excerpts from a few sessions with Joyce that I described at the beginning of chapter two. I noted there that I presented them not as a sterling example of therapeutic technique, but because the material served well to illustrate in dramatic form some characteristics of the zero process. For purposes of argument, however, I would now like to take a look at what might have been wrong with my clinical work. I questioned Joyce about the possible meaning of her reactions. Even when she said, "I feel you're pushing me. You're pulling me into this, into looking at this, but it's not good," I still kept at it. I have presented this example at a number of meetings, and each time clinicians have gotten up and said that I was enacting the trauma with Joyce, and that I should have pulled back and that my interventions were detrimental. I agreed with the idea of enactment, and I didn't suggest that what I did was a fine example of technique. But I did note that Joyce had been in analysis and therapy for many years at the time of these sessions, and that she had managed to work through some very difficult childhood traumas. And, what to me seemed most significant, Joyce had in the long run suffered no ill effects from the piece of work, and in fact had benefited quite a bit. Even in the short run, while the sessions described were ongoing, Joyce was able to carry on with her regular life.

Despite what I said, questioners persisted, noting that perhaps this type of thing may work in expert hands, but that it was dangerous to set it up as a way to approach trauma. Less experienced therapists may model themselves on this approach and hurt their patients. While in one way I appreciated the complement of being considered such an expert, from another angle I felt these comments put this kind of exploration of trauma not as part of regular therapeutic technique, but rather as something extraordinary. Certainly the sessions with Joyce were dramatic, and were not the norm in her therapy. But with many patients there are some sessions of great intensity, although often not quite so dramatic as Joyce's. I have given some examples with Peggy and Cordelia. Each of these involved the living out of zero process memories, often quite strongly.

In the case of people with borderline disorders, and/or with severe developmental interference in the building of their inner structure, when one opens up a true trauma, such as a rape, the person will usually get so overwhelmed that they experience an uncontrolled regression. The sort of work I did with Joyce or some of the other examples that I have presented, would be more difficult with such patients. In their case it may often be better to work on stabilization, avoiding going too deeply into major traumas. In borderline disorders one would concentrate on present day difficulties with building up stable self and object images, with integrating "good" and "bad" self and object representations, with affect modulation, and with differentiating fantasy from reality, among many other ego difficulties. In those with other sorts of developmental interference work on structural difficulties, and often their connection with past chronic situations that interfered with their development (deprivation, instability, threat, overgratification, etc.), will need attention first. If this work goes well, one may then be in a position to approach traumas, but even then one has to tread carefully and slowly, being ready to work on other dynamics. The sort of confrontation of avoidance of trauma that is helpful in a better functioning patient would not be so for such patients, certainly not before much preparatory work. On the other hand it would greatly hinder the therapy of trauma in a more neurotic patient if one withdrew back to trying to strengthen their ego each time they started to feel overwhelmed while exploring traumatic memories. In doing this one would be mistaking their feelings that they were falling to pieces or too weak, for reports about the present state of their capacities, rather than recognizing them as zero process memories from their trauma.

This difference is a chance to make an important distinction between mental contents and mental dynamics. This distinction is a key component of the ego psychological point of view while it is not as important, or even seen as a mirage, in some other theories. As an example, we could take Joyce's reactions during the sessions that I described. While she did not state it explicitly, her very powerful reactions, and what she did say, suggested that she felt that the work was beyond her capacities. To repeat a part of the clinical material: as I was asking her about the details of what happened, I noted that Joyce moaned, "Nooo, Nooo. You're pulling me and pushing me now. It's not good."

"So it feels like it's now?" I said.

"It is now. You're just pushing me too hard and I can't breathe. There's a burning in my throat. It hurts a lot."

Despite her powerful feelings that the emerging memories were beyond her capacities to handle, the work did actually help Joyce and proved not to be beyond her capacities. It was clear from the way the reliving unfolded that the feeling of being overwhelmed and of falling apart were zero process memories. These feelings were a content of the mind, in this case a piece of the past reality of the rape that was unprocessed and experienced as a feeling in the present. The key thing is that a feeling of falling apart, even an extremely intense one, cannot automatically be equated with the person's mind actually falling to pieces. Sometimes these feelings seem to have an extra level of intensity and reality, which makes us suspect they really are internal perceptions of a mind falling to pieces. In some cases this is true. But the theory of the zero process tells us that it could also be a reality from another time, not recognized as such by the patient, but rather experienced as a present reality.

When these feelings are truly zero process memories, and the patient is not compromised in other ways, it is helpful to interpret them histori-cally. Such an interpretation might be, "I wonder if this feeling of being so small and weak and unable to manage is really a memory of your mental state when the trauma was ongoing. It's a memory masquerading as a present experience." This is a version of an interpretation of the zero process that has quite general applicability, in which one points out that a present experience is actually a form of memory. Another good example of a zero process memory that looks similar to borderline functioning was given by Peggy, my patient with the mother who suffered from paranoid schizophrenia. Peggy would often say that she felt alone, and that no one really cared for her or loved her, in a matter of fact manner, as if stating an obvious reality—which confusingly contradicted her de-scriptions of all the people she met and meaningful conversations she had with them. Here too, given all that had emerged about her early history, I said to her, "I wonder if the reason that this feeling of being completely alone and that no one loves you feels so real, is because it is real. It's a memory of real situations in your past with your mother, appearing now as a present day experience." These sorts of interventions led to Peggy described how she had always lived at two levels, with the darkness and aloneness down below, and brightness and connection above. She connected it to her treatment by her psychopathic husband as well. Rather than becoming overwhelmed by such interventions, she almost always felt much better and less depressed.

While her complaints of aloneness and not being loved were similar to what we might hear from someone with borderline dynamics, it was easy enough to tell by Peggy's history, her general presentation, and her be-haviour in therapy, including her stable capacity to relate to me and form a very good connection over many years, that she did not suffer from a borderline disorder. In cases at one extreme, such as Peggy who was clearly a well functioning and integrated person, or the other extreme such as patients with major instability, making the distinction is rela-tively easy. In others, differentiating the two conditions is not so easy, for various reasons. The level of the borderline deficit may be relatively low, or in a person with reasonable ego capacities, the particular post-traumatic reactions may have so taken over their life that they may on superficial observation appear to have a pervasive personality disorder with chronic instability, even though what is really going on is the living out of traumatic memories. In the end, if one keeps an open mind, the further course of therapy usually makes the situation clear. A not un-common situation is a serious trauma taking place at a time when the child or adolescent is in a psychological situation similar to borderline or other

serious disorder. I have seen patients with traumas during the rap-
prochement phase (about one and a half years of age) and early adolescence, both times in which there is an instability of affects and self/other
boundaries, who at times could looked not just disturbed, but disturbed in
a specifically borderline way. They were not. One part of them was living
in a borderline reality from the time of the trauma. (For an example of this
type of situation, see my discussion below, in this section, of a patient
whose therapy is described in a 2019 article by Ignês Sodré.)

People with personality disorders are rather quick to accept comments
about possible traumas, generally being less resistant to them than more
neurotic individuals. This has two causes: they have a strong tendency to
externalize, especially negative feelings, and they have weakened repressions. These act in concert. Actual traumas are not as securely repressed and defended against and these, as well as situations that may
not have been traumatic, are used as screens upon which to project
scenes of inner turmoil and devastation that are a product, as are the
weak repressions, of difficulties with stabilizing emotional and drive
investments. It is a common experience to feel early on with many not so
severe borderline patients that one is really getting somewhere, as central
traumas and deprivations are quickly brought into view. There can be a
feeling of excitement that mirrors the patient's living out of the positive
side of split feelings. But somehow things never quite come together. The
patient keeps talking of the trauma—often one trauma or depriving relationship will be felt as the explanation for everything. But there is no
deepening of the feelings or fleshing out of details from the trauma, as
happened with patients such as Peggy or Cordelia, and there is also not the
same exposing of the web of connections from the trauma to other traumas
and emotional conflicts. This is also true for these emotional conflicts, for
instance conflicts over envy and aggression related to siblings, or oedipal
rivalry. These can come up quite dramatically and against less resistance
than in more neurotic patients, but the work doesn't deepen, nor do the
connections with other issues emerge in workable ways. The most fundamental cause of this is the inability to sublimate, which leads to the weak
repressions and lessened synthetic abilities, but also to intense investments
in various explanations for the person's troubles. These investments lead to
great excitement but lack stability and nuance and modulation, demonstrating that the deepening of the work, as with the deepening of the
personality, requires neutralization and sublimation of basic drives.

Let's approach the comparison of trauma with other forms of causation
and other problems from another angle—that of the transference. We
could use the ideas presented so far about trauma and the zero process in
such an endeavour. I would distinguish three broad forms of transference: the standard displacement transference across a repression barrier,
such as Peggy's father transference onto me; projective identifications

such as L's, which replace a crumbling repression by putting pieces of the person's mind into the other; and zero process transferences such as Joyce had in an extreme form during her reliving. This is certainly not the only way to divide up transferences (for instance Kernberg (2019) presents a classification based on an object relations point of view), but it does not contradict other classifications. It is relatively simple, and is based on the elemental underlying form of mental functioning at work in each case.

The classical transference that Freud described was based on a number of characteristics of primary process, including displacement, and the precedence of fantasy over reality, in interaction with the defensive and modulatory capacities of the secondary process. Cordelia unconsciously displaced her attachment, feelings, and Oedipal wishes and conflicts from her father, and her mother, onto me. This was a transference across a repression barrier in that the most powerful memories and wishes were held in check by repression, so that what emerged grew slowly in strength as the therapeutic regression took hold. The feelings rarely and only temporarily flooded out the real relationship between Cordelia and me (for instance at times when she became very angry at me), and thus their historical roots could be explored and unpacked and made conscious. I have not detailed this part of our therapy together, as I have concentrated on Cordelia's traumas, but the analytic literature is full of detailed descriptions of such transferences. This transference has characteristics of both the primary process (displacement, condensation—for instance in Cordelia's case, between feelings for her mother and father, and from different points in her childhood—lack of distinction between fantasy and reality, etc.) and the secondary process (control and modulation of the regression, selective repression).

Projective identification, as I described it previously, involves the substantial and not just temporary or partial weakening of primal repressions, so that the characteristics of the primary process flood out realistic aspects of the relationship, as happened for instance in L's reactions to me. Many characteristics of the primary process that are usually held in check by repression and modified by the more reality oriented secondary process in neurotic transferences, come to the fore and define projective identification. These include the lack of integration between various emotional trends such as love and hate, and the instability and lack of permanence of emotional investments. I have described my view of the dynamics of borderline disorders and projective identification in some detail in the last chapter. Here I will compare them at the clinical level to the presentation and treatment of the zero process.

I was pulled into a certain type of friendly relationship with Cordelia that mirrored her early one with her father, and an even earlier one with her mother, but I was not pulled into her mind. I did not disappear into her mind as I became a piece of her, as I did with my patient L, where in the sessions described I became the embodiment of her sadistic wishes and vindictive feelings. Intense eruptions of zero process memories, such as I described with Joyce, can look superficially similar to the sort of powerful interactions of projective identification, but they are different in their inner structure. In zero process transferences, rather than being trapped in the patient's mind, one is trapped in their past reality. While the zero process outbursts can be jarring at times, they do not invade the therapist's mind to nearly the same extent. I could see that Joyce was scared of me, but I didn't feel like a scary and bad person, as I did with L. And the effects of the eruption in the case of trauma disappear as quickly as they appear. The way in which certain induced feelings last for hours or days in cases of strong projective identifications is characteristic of, and diagnostic of, the defense. By contrast, the manner in which the therapist gets caught up in traumatic reliving bears many of the hallmarks of the zero process. It comes on suddenly and disappears just as suddenly, in the classic manner of zero process memories. I was not left with the feelings that Joyce's reliving stirred up in me for long afterwards, as I was with L's accusations against me. In this, I believe the therapist mirrors the dissociated nature of the zero process, which is powerfully present and then just as powerfully not present.

Because the transferences of borderlines and neurotics are both at bottom related to the functioning of the primary process, they are more closely related to each other in their deepest nature than they are to zero process transferences. I have until now stressed the differences between neurotic dynamics and borderline ones, and between projective identification and classical transferences, but if we take a few steps further back and take a broader view, they share similarities when compared to zero process transferences, due to this similar derivation from the workings of the primary process. There is a similar manner in which the therapist's inner world gets caught up in the inner world of the patient—it just does so in a much more modulated and slower, and somewhat more hidden, manner in the case of neurotic transferences such as Cordelia's, as compared to L's projective identifications.

In the case of a zero process transference, rather than invasion of the therapy and therapist by internal drives and affects, and internalized conflicts and overwhelming situations from the past, one is faced with an invasion from the outside, by an external past reality. One could object that after all, these past realities are memories inside the patient's mind, and are not external at all, and not real. This is not untrue. But the central argument of this book, from the discussion of differences between memory and perception, to the elucidation of how things only happen once they are fully constructed, and how they otherwise remain psychologically as immediate perceptual realities, to the detailed discussions of the breakdown of the first-order construction of reality during the traumatic process, has led to this important clinical point: *the zero process appears in therapy and analysis not as an inner psychological reality, but as the intrusion of a piece of external reality, with all the characteristics of external reality, and it is in this that it differs quite thoroughly from the intrusions of inner reality we see in projective identifications and in neurotic transferences.*

I have already noted the way in which zero process memories do not invade the therapist's mind in the same manner as other transferences. This is not to say that the therapist is not effected by the patient's zero process memories, but they are effected in some very peculiar ways. I tended to forget and dismiss the importance of Cordelia's early traumas, just as she did. Just as it is for the patient, the therapist may have little awareness of what certain actions or reactions mean, and then in a flash, they will know. One may be tempted to be suspicious of these pieces of sudden knowledge, or alternatively to see in them some special force at work, perhaps a mystical connection between two people. But there is a perfectly rational explanation for the appearance of this knowledge. The patient lives in two realities, only one of which they are aware of at most times. Through various and many subtle and not so subtle reactions on the patient's part, we are informed of their other reality. We use our basic observational and empathic capacities to gather this information, and we use our basic capacity to construct reality from these bits and pieces—a capacity that we use every minute of every day—to construct the patient's past traumatic reality from the bits and pieces we intuit from the patient. This information gathering and constructing is done unconsciously, and the outcome at times becomes conscious in what is experienced as a flash of insight.

It is useful to learn the difference between this way of gaining awareness of our patient's traumatic realities, and other sorts of intuitions that we have about their emotional lives and past. When we listen with evenly hovering attention, trying to relax and allow ourselves to tune in to our patient's unconscious, we pick up on clues from their tone, derivatives, feelings, etc., about the patient's (primary process) unconscious, that we read with our own unconscious. Much has been written about this, from Freud's early descriptions to the present. We resonate with certain feelings and internalizations of early relationships, become aware of aspects of the patient's past and unconscious through empathic resonance, and enact some of this with them. My experience has been, both as a clinician and a supervisor, that this differs fundamentally from what was described above about the manner in which we become aware of unprocessed traumas. In terms of treating trauma, becoming aware of how the counter resistance of avoidance feels in us, and of how it feels when we unconsciously construct the unprocessed traumas of our patients, can serve as invaluable guides in telling us where dwells the zero process, in helping us to make out its contents, and in helping us also to know when things that may superficially look like trauma are something else entirely.

The manner in which we pick up on the patient's zero process memories mirrors the manner in which children do so with parents and grandparents. It is the manner in which trauma is passed down through the generations. Thus a proper understanding of these dynamics promises to have quite wide application. The zero process is a second reality. It is a frozen set of moments. We could say the zero process is a "preconstruction phase" of the building of reality, when all the building materials are still just lying around, waiting to be put together. When we have flashes of what these traumas are, we have intuitively become aware of some of these pieces and have quickly and unconsciously put a part of the traumatic reality together. This constructional activity is a normal part of our mind's functioning. We have to constantly perform this construction in order to properly perceive reality. And so, once we sense the pieces of someone else's reality lying around, we quite naturally turn our activity on them. The child of traumatized relatives does the same thing. Although they often do not consciously become aware of this second reality that they construct, their thoughts and feelings and actions are affected by it.

Having made these comments with regard to differentiating the manner in which the zero process impinges on the therapy, compared to other phenomena, it may perhaps be helpful to give an example from recent literature to make a few points about the how these various modes of functioning are differentiated at times, and become tangled up at others, in present day psychoanalytic theory and practice. In the Centenary Special Issue of the International Journal of Psychoanalysis there is a section on trauma with a number of articles. In one of these articles, Ignês Sodré (2019) describes her work with a woman, Alicia, who changes the topic when uncomfortable and in other ways denies realities. She has a whole split off fantasy life, of sexual relations with women, based on women she meets, that she can go into and out of quickly, and that runs in parallel with her regular heterosexual life. Alicia lives in these two worlds. Sodré conceptualizes what is going on using Freud's idea of splitting of the ego, and builds on this Freudian conceptualization. She develops a distinction between different dynamics and forms of functioning similar to the one I have developed in this book: the repressed that returns (I would say neurotic treatment of the primary process), which she describes as mobile; secondly the version of the repressed which appears more alien to the person when they have split it off and projected it (projective identification); and finally the dissociated part of the mind, that is always there on another track, which they can jump onto or off from (what I would call the zero process).

My hope is that by using a clearly written clinical article from the literature, readers can refer if they wish to the original with regard to the points I am making. Sodré describes two sets of traumas that emerged from Alicia's reactions and transferences, one beginning from when she was one month old and her parents would go on business trips and leave her with a favourite and very loving and doting relative, "Auntie" (the much younger sister of the patient's maternal grandmother). The second trauma was the parents' disintegrating marriage and eventual divorce when Alicia was five, with her father becoming less connected to her psychologically, and her mother becoming so depressed that Auntie had to look after both patient and mother. Sodré discusses the clinical progress of the case, as well as using it to discuss different dynamic issues. She sees, as I said, that there is a set of dissociated reactions and internal objects and fantasies related to these traumas that differ from more regular objects and fantasies. But she approaches this area of post-traumatic functioning largely with the concepts that her theory uses to understand other aspects of the unconscious. In her case, this is Kleinian object relations theory.

Alicia has a few serious outbursts, quite unexpectedly and seemingly unpredictably. I will quote Sodré's description of the one of these: "The next day she arrived visibly disturbed and withdrawn, and didn't speak for a long time. Eventually she said she had almost not come today because of my horrible cruelty: I had said 'in touch' although I never touch her, never give a hug. This was a more violent than usual transformation after the end of the session—crossing the threshold between my room and outside, she found herself in a murderous world; she had seriously considered ending the analysis. This had a different quality from the melancholic scenario of abandonment; for the first time I felt she was frightened of me. Gradually it became clear that she 'knew,' with delusional conviction, that when she left each session she disappeared from my mind, ceasing to exist. In contrast, she felt compelled to think of me all the time, in a disturbing way. This new, persecuting version of a parallel continuous story was linked to what she experienced as the bizarreness of the analytic structure, and heralded the appearance, in the transference and countertransference, of a concretely experienced Schizoid Object with a bizarre mind." (pp. 1178–1179.)

This reaction is conceptualized by Sodré as having to do with the behaviour of internal objects, attacking and doing other things that internal objects do, even if in a strange and different manner. Of course with just this one vignette, things could be interpreted in many ways. It certainly could be an outburst similar to what I described with my patient L, involving projective identification. The content of this, of not being kept in mind, seems a direct description of the weak object constancy, and weak self constancy, that is at the heart of borderline disorders and that seems to be projected onto the analyst. And the absolute certainty is something we see with eruptions of the primary process leading to projective identification—the certainty surpasses normal certainty, and feels delusional. But the larger context makes it clear, as the author notes, that this is not a borderline or psychotic patient. Sodré tries to deal with the presence of these borderline-like reactions by the idea of splitting of the ego, suggesting that in one side of this split does have a delusional denial of reality, and that Alicia uses this fact to protect the belief that she can change reality and cling to the perfect mother.

In seeking to understand these split off areas of strange, concrete, unsymbolized functioning using modified concepts from existing theories, such as paranoid schizoid functioning and delusional thinking, Sodré can't quite let go of the ideas that served her in other situations. This is generally the case for many theorists, from the object relations, Freudian, intersubjective, and other schools as well. Sodré (p. 1174) states that a "striking thing about Alicia was how her capacity for ordinarily neurotic object relations, with the normal oscillation between depressive and paranoid-schizoid positions – the fluidity between aspects of the self of different stages of development and oscillating also between predominantly loving and predominantly aggressive emotions – was present and real in the analysis; I was impressed by her capacity for insight. This was surprising considering the seriousness of the dissociation and of the splitting of her ego; the split-off part of the self was experienced, almost, as another self." This only seems surprising to the author because she is using ideas related to delusion and psychosis, and thus feels Alicia must be quite disturbed, although she is a clear eyed enough observer to see that this is not the case.

To my mind, the observations are not so much surprising as diagnostic. They tell us that Alicia is a person with good general ego functioning who suffers from zero process memories, just as Joyce and Peggy did. One might object that the author in fact says exactly this. This is true, but she sees these post-traumatic memories as something like other problems, only perhaps more extreme than borderline problems, and more sequestered and compartmentalized than regular psychotic ones. She herself sees that this can't be completely true but, to repeat myself, is unwilling to understand the traumatic memories completely on their own terms. She begins to fashion concepts to comprehend them, but to my reading can't quite go all the way in this. This is a good illustration of a general situation within psychoanalytic theorizing on trauma. This theoretical position has clinical consequences. From this position, one will analyze the movements and nature of the inner objects, and the manner in which they play out in the transference and countertransference, as one would with other dynamics. As examples, Sodré interprets that Alicia feels that she is responsible for her parents' marriage breakup, and works on what she sees as the different internal mothers from the traumas playing out in the analytic relationship.

For this approach, one will have lots of material. The zero process memories connect with all sorts of emotional conflicts and other issues, and so these are present in relation to the trauma and connected to the areas of split off zero process functioning. As an example, I described how the illness and death of Cordelia's mother had become entangled with her reactions to the birth of her two siblings, including feeling abandoned and angry at her mother, as well as with complex Oedipal conflicts, and also with difficulties with her step mother from later childhood and adolescence. Work on these issues can be quite useful, will often take up much of the therapy time, and lead to positive changes. But only up to a point. It was only as we fully accessed and analyzed the zero process memories that the various conflicts, deprivations, and chronic stresses had become attached to, that these other dynamics and issues were able to be processed.

In terms of this example from the literature, one might argue that after all the analyst was analyzing her patient's traumas. That is mainly what she presents. In a short paper it would be impossible for her to present even the main parts of the clinical work of an analysis, so that what I have to say on this matter should not be taken as a commentary or criticism of Sodré's work in particular, but rather as a more general commentary on difficulties with modern techniques, and on what the theory of the zero process can add to them. Sodré's patient Alicia has an intense reaction in which she was certain that her analyst will forget her completely. Sodré calls this a delusion, but given the way it emerges, and the patient's other characteristics, I have argued that it is a zero process memory, even though it bears a resemblance to borderline reactions. To analyze it as a "reliving" of a past trauma, within the relationship, does not fully address this. To begin with, I would give basic zero process interpretations, such as, "what happened after the session, and the certainty about me forgetting you is, I think, a memory. It's not labelled as a memory, but I think it is a memory of what happened to you a number of times in your early childhood."

This might seem a subtle difference, to call it a memory rather than a reliving. But it is an acknowledgment that this is the form in which the unprocessed parts of the trauma now live. To suggest that the patient is reliving a memory of their past paints a picture of something like a strong regular memory, that is now brought to life and relived. But the truly unprocessed parts of the trauma only live on as present and future experiences, and it is better to name them as such and deal with them as such. This is not about intellectual correctness, but clinical power. I have found that when things are phrased in this way, further traumatic memories emerge and the therapy moves forward much more quickly.

In the case of any serious trauma with zero process memories, one is exploring not the patient's inner mind, but rather one of the realities that they live with and in. One needs to address them as such. One needs to talk to the patient about how they live in two, and sometimes more, realities. One needs to tell them that the traumatic incidents have shattered into a hundred pieces of memory and feeling and thought, and that these have been scattered in the present and future, embedded in other things. Of course one does not have to say exactly these things, but one does need to address the traumatic memories directly, not treating them like regular memories, or fantasies, or regular internal objects, or emotional conflicts over childhood sexual wishes and aggression, or attachment issues, or personality disorders. The shards from the shattered traumatic incidents can embed in these things, and they can also look like these things as they freeze moments in time, such as Alicia's weak object constancy as an abandoned young child, that relate to these issues. But the zero process memories are none of these things, and only by addressing them on their own terms can we truly free the patient from their hold.

The first steps in analyzing the zero process is being able to spot it and to name it as such, first saying that it may have something to do with the past trauma, and then making basic zero process interpretations about the reactions being memories. One should discuss with the patient the dissociation they are experiencing and nature of traumatic memories. The use of intellectual discussions as a defense in some circumstances does not mean that they are not needed as a scaffolding for the construction of the unconstructed parts of the past trauma when dealing with the zero process. Usually once one starts this conversation, the patient opens up about this separate world that they have been living with and in. Patients usually experience it as a great relief to be able to put words to it, as Peggy did when she started to talk of the "dark underbelly" that she had lived with "all my life—I can't remember when I didn't have it." We then traced its origins in the bizarre and sometimes genuinely scary experiences with her paranoid schizophrenic mother, and then how similar experiences with her abusive psychopathic husband also ended up in this underbelly.

Providing the scaffolding gives the structure and narrative, but one needs also to put the pieces together. This is the construction of the trauma from the zero process bits and pieces. This construction has often been confused with the reconstruction of the past that is important (and in some quarters much neglected) in analyzing emotional conflicts, deprivation, and stresses. In these later cases, there are repressed and denied, but constructed, memories, that have to be unearthed, and usually synthesized and integrated with the person's life narrative for the first time. But they do not need to be constructed for the first time, as does the zero process core of a trauma. Between these two extremes are partial cases, of chronic stresses and less severe traumas, where some aspects of higher level construction, such as being put in a narrative and understood as to their meaning, have not been performed, but they are at least partially constructed. The analysis of these various aspects of people's overwhelming and unprocessed realities is the topic of the next section.

The Central Post-Traumatic Complex

In the section on "fixation to trauma" in chapter one, I mentioned Furst's (1978) idea of bland trauma, and gave an example of a bland trauma of one of my patients who had been involved in a car accident. In this type of trauma zero process memories are formed from an overwhelming incident, but over the ensuing days and weeks and months processing of the traumatic memories in dreams and reliving seems to go to completion, and the person is freed from any further effects of the incident. The fact that some traumas are bland traumas tells us a few things of interest for the treatment of trauma. It tells us that there already exists a normal and relatively automatic process, analogous to the mourning process with loss, that evokes the zero process memories and allows them to be dealt with in a manner that does away with their hold on the person and on their present and future. It tells us that intervening right after a trauma in order to get the person to talk about what has happened and process it consciously will not always have positive results, as it may interfere with relatively automatic and unconscious processing. In the early stages it is probably best to provide comfort, and space and time for the person to recover, and to talk if they wish, just as one would in the case of somebody who has lost someone. In both of these situations people generally realize that it is best to create conditions of safety and support, and ritual and structure, which allow for the processing of the trauma and/or for the mourning process to proceed to completion.

If all traumas were bland traumas, there would be no need for trauma therapy. The descriptor bland does not mean that such traumas are boring or have no excitement, but rather than they have no admixture of anything else, by analogy with food that has no spices or other flavourings added. Bland traumas are traumas pure and simple. It is the admixtures that interfere with the automatic post-traumatic processing, and that thus necessitate trauma therapy. Trauma therapy essentially involves identifying and neutralizing these admixtures to enough of an extent that the usual automatic processing of the zero process memories can finally take place.

One complicating factor can be the intensity of the trauma, which leads both to much more powerful primary dissociation of the zero process memories, and to such overwhelming feelings when the curative reliving starts, that the person avoids the reliving through various means, including by further dissociations. In order to set the natural curative process going again, one needs to counter the avoidance and dissociation. The techniques and therapies I discussed at the start of this chapter attempt to break through the dissociation by approaching the zero process memories on their own terms (sensorimotor therapy, art therapy, dance/movement therapy) and/or by attempting to calm the overstimulation so that it does not lead to a shutdown of reintegration (EMDR, hypnosis). Many aspects of more regular dynamic therapy for trauma involve measures designed to achieve the same ends, including providing support and containment, and taking smaller bits of the trauma to analyze.

There are other things that can hinder the natural healing processes. An unfortunately quite common situation involves further traumas, following one after the other, and/or a chronic state of instability in the environment, often the family, even if it doesn't always reach traumatic intensity. In these situations the person will quite naturally shut down the disruption that comes from processing previous traumas, as they try to manage the present situation. Lack of emotional support, or the withdrawal of it in relation especially to the traumas (such as denial of sexual abuse by the non-abusing parent), will have similar effects, as the person is not afforded the space and time to do the work of processing. Situations of childhood sexual or physical abuse within families often involve both the factors of trauma repetition and partial or total lack of interpersonal support.

Another major reason for the fixation of a trauma is that it becomes embroiled with conflict dynamics. This is a fixation that works in both directions, as a trauma becoming connected with a major conflict is likely to make that conflict harder to resolve, even as this connection also fixates the trauma. With ongoing traumatization and stress, and with the connection of the trauma to other conflicts and issues, various defenses are brought into play to keep the zero process drive to relive the trauma at bay. These include all of the well known defenses that have been studied for over a century: denial, repression, regression, and obsessional defenses such as reaction formation and isolation of affect. Shengold (1988, 1989) has described in detail how anal/obsessive defenses are used after trauma to control overwhelming feelings, at the cost of a great narrowing of the person's emotional life. I have said most of what I have to say about these various defenses earlier in this book (see for instance the sections "repression" and "dissociation" in chapter three), in the case presentations, and in my previous book (2009), which explored the topic of defenses in detail.

The more original contribution to the treatment of trauma that I have to offer at this point relates to the analysis of what I have called zero process drive/defense conflicts. An understanding of the nature of these conflicts is, I think, a major addition that zero process theory can make both to trauma theory, and to clinical practice. I have outlined most of the theoretical aspects of zero process defenses in previous chapters, especially in different sections of chapter three: in the section on "The Zero Process Drive" I outlined the basic nature of this drive that continuously pushes for the living out of the traumatic zero process memories as actualities; and in the sections on "Dissociation," "Zero Process Denial and Temporal Shifting," and "Dissociative Identity Disorder and Splitting of the Identity," I described the nature of various zero process defenses that oppose this drive and attempt to keep it at bay or redirect it. At this point I would like to describe a basic post-traumatic complex of zero process defenses that regularly forms after trauma. It includes a conjunction of different processes I have described: dissociation, zero process denial, temporal shifting, and some version of splitting of the identity.

To set the stage for my description of how these defenses work in concert to hold the traumatic memories at bay even as they are also given some displaced expression, I will summarize some of what I have said previously. I described both zero process denial and temporal shifting as using the "not yet happened" nature of zero process memories for defensive purposes. I described how treating the zero process memories as realities led to good results clinically. I will repeat an example I gave in relation to the defense of temporal shifting that addresses this issue of treating the traumatic memories as present day realities. I noted that Cordelia always lived with a future in which someone died and she was left abandoned. She lived at the point just before the full impact of the trauma, when there was a chance to still save her mother. And she rushed to help and treat those that she saw as in danger. I noted that a non zero process interpretation might be something like, "what you're afraid will happen to yourself or the people you rush to help is what happened to your mother." This treats Cordelia's fear as a kind of learned response from the past, informing fears of the future, or perhaps, in a more analytic sense, it could be seen as a wish and/or fantasy about what might happen to these people, as she might have wished or feared it with her mother. But this interpretation is inaccurate. What lived in Cordelia's future was neither a memory of the past projected into the future, nor a fantasy. Thus, what I said to Cordelia was, "your mother's death hasn't yet happened to you. It remains in your future and you keep it there to keep open the possibility that it will all turn out differently." I also said, "the loss of your mother has crowded out many more realistic possibilities in your future, as it has come to live there, and the time just before that loss has come to dominate your present."

It is an intrinsic characteristic of what I will call the **central post-traumatic complex** that the traumatized person lives, as Cordelia did, at the point just before the full force of the trauma hit, and thus just before their mind was shattered. Often, the usual processing of the trauma will have been put off as further traumas occurred, or because of the lack of support and the size of the trauma. This perfectly reasonable need to put off processing because of circumstances is then extended indefinitely, for defensive reasons. For this purpose the immediate, "just happening" nature of the zero process is used. The seeming repetitions of traumas are rarely simple expressions of a repetition compulsion, but are rather the product of zero process drive/defense conflicts. They are compromise formations. The zero process drive pushes for repetitious reliving— although we should more accurately say that this drive pushes for repetition as part of the belated processing and mastery of the trauma. A pure expression of the drive would not lead to endless repetition. The "repetition compulsion" as we have come to know it, as a monotonously repeating set of feelings and experiences and actions, is usually a product of the push of the zero process drive modified by zero process defenses. Some part of the repetition of extreme traumatization may be an exception, but I am describing these zero process drive/defense conflicts because it is important clinically, I feel, to not immediately assume an irreducible repetition compulsion before trying to analyze the sorts of dynamics I have described, and will describe further below.

A clinical point worth emphasizing is that the patient's strong feeling that to re-experience the trauma is beyond their capacities is often not a true self assessment, but rather part of the central post-traumatic complex: it involves living a past reality as a present one, of not being able to handle and process the trauma, as a way of fending off the zero process drive to process the trauma. A clear understanding of the nature of this defense is crucial for any approach to trauma, as without it the therapist often ends up circling around the trauma, analyzing related themes, sometimes approaching the core traumatic memories gingerly, and then pulling back in the face of a zero process defense that they mistake for a patient's inability to go further.

But what if the patient really is not ready and you push them, based on mistaken ideas? I would say there are risks on both sides, and one needs to be clear on what they are, which depends not just on one intervention but on the whole course of a therapy and how it is conducted. There is usually very little to be gained, and much to be lost, in putting off interpretation of defenses such as reluctance and avoidance and of the zero process defensive complex. Of course before interpreting one first gets a therapy going, establishing trust and safety and a reasonable alliance, as you and the patient get to know each other and the patient tells their story and begins to form transferences. I am not suggesting simply pushing a patient in relation to their traumas, but rather interpreting specific defenses. One might say, "I wonder if your feeling that this will overwhelm you and destroy you, if you go further in thinking about it, is actually a memory of what it was like when the trauma was at its height?" As with any interpretation of a defense, a denial doesn't mean you are on the wrong track, any more than assent by the patient means that you are on the right one. It all depends on what comes after. In any case an interpretation like this is part of a process, and is designed to help this process move along and deepen. Done in the right manner, there is not much danger in making it—if one is wrong, one risks disagreement, and perhaps anger or regression, but these too will be clarifying about the patient's situation. On the other hand not making the interpretation over extended periods of time risks the danger of a therapy, unfortunately an all too common situation, going on for years or even decades in a quasi-stalemated position as one circles around possible traumas.

I believe, having experienced it personally and seen it in many others, that a basic countertransference response in the face of trauma is avoidance and minimization, leading to delay in approaching the trauma on the part of the therapist. Related to the response of delaying inter-pretation and exploration of the trauma is a disbelief in the availability of various forms of memory, but especially perceptual and semantic (knowledge) memories, related to the trauma. If these memories are not approached and unearthed from behind various defenses and in the various places they are hiding, such as the future, the analysis of the trauma can become truly chaotic and overwhelming. I want to be clear about what I am asserting. I am not suggesting that every disbelief or reluctance on the part of a therapist is a countertransference resistance, nor that every memory that a patient brings forward has to be believed as true rather than being interrogated and analyzed. Rather, I am describing a common countertransference response to the emergence of material related to serious trauma of a patient. One can use this response as a guide in further work. Awareness of it alerts one to dissociated trauma in the patient and can help one come up with useful interventions.

Understanding the nature of zero process defenses and how they form the central post-traumatic complex allows us to crack open what otherwise appears as a simple compulsion to repeat the trauma. Merely pointing out this repetition to the patient does not in general lead to any change. But analyzing the zero process dynamics holding it in place often does. I have found that things really open up with interpretations of zero process de-fenses such as zero process denial and temporal shifting, and of the various zero process memories hidden in plain sight in the patient's present day reactions and their fears and other expectations related to the future. If one suspects that a reaction is one of these memories, it is usually worthwhile interpreting, and seeing what comes up, always being open to the possi-bility that the reaction is not the memory you suspected it to be.

The future often contains a rich trove of memories, if one looks carefully and persistently enough. A first step can be to inquire into the specific contents of phobic fears or other expectations. I have found that simply inquiring in more detail about specific ideas or fears for the future can give one an idea about details of a person's trauma. Often patients will be resistant, wanting to describe their fear as simply "abandonment fear," or "attachment problems." But if one persists in asking how they concretely picture it, one is often rewarded by details of the trauma, living in the future. The reluctance to go into details is also telling, reluctance and avoidance being characteristic reactions to traumatic memories.

Any of the patients I have presented, and I would argue any of your patients, if you happen to be a clinician, will prove to have many of the details of their serious traumas hiding in plain sight, in their future. I have found it to be helpful to show an interest in the details of these fears or other feelings about the future rather than argue against them or insist that they belong to the past. In fact often the patient themselves will try to dismiss the ideas about the future as unrealistic, saying that they have to get over them by realizing how irrational they are. Faced with this, I usually insist that there is something important in these ideas of the future, and that the very fact that the patient is so certain of them is no reason to try to fight them. In fact, this certainty itself is a sign. One can usually only be so certain, I say, about what has happened in the past. This type of certainty marks these ideas out as memories, and they may have a lot to tell us if we inquire into them. (Of course absolute certainty and a lack of negation are also characteristics of the primary process, so the point I make here is for purposes of interpretation—the fact that someone is certain of a future fear is not proof that it comes from a trauma. Usually phobic fears involve zero process memories and primary process fantasies bound tightly together.)

The final elements of the central post-traumatic complex are dynamics and structures with similarities to those of DID, that I have described as a product of splitting of the identity. I believe that these identities are used to control the zero process drive that pushes for repetition. Just as in traditional drive/defense conflicts primal repression does the heavy lifting of keeping the push of the drive at bay, while denials and other defenses play a central role in dealing with memories and fantasies, so too in the case of trauma splitting of the identity does basic work in holding the push of zero process drive at bay, and temporal shifting and similar defenses work to keep the zero process memories out of awareness by depositing them in the future, denying them, etc. I find many analysts who are open to ideas such as the dynamics of temporal shifting, draw the line at taking alters and alter-like phenomena seriously enough to address them directly as separate entities. This is felt as abandoning our hard won understanding of the inner world of fantasies and wishes and defenses, as well as our sophisticated understanding of the formations of internal objects as representations that are really memory/fantasy complexes imbued with affects from recurring early interactions and traumas.

I have presented my ideas about the nature of alters and DID phenomena, as the most elaborated outcome of the basic post-traumatic defense of splitting of the identity, at length in the section "Dissociative Identity Disorder and Splitting of the Identity" at the end of chapter three. Because of the resistance of many psychoanalysts to these ideas, I wanted to present detailed enough clinical material and comprehensive enough conceptual/theoretical arguments in relation to these topics so that they, including the reality of the alters, could be seen as understandable outcomes of serious trauma. An understanding of these dynamics is relevant not just for the special case of DID, but for all other serious traumas. Everyone who has had serious trauma has alter-like split off entities: aspects of identity wrapped around key powerful zero process memories, animated by the zero process drive, that behave as partially independent canters of initiative.

Many therapies posit such entities as the inner child or inner parent, and psychoanalysis posits internal objects and introjects. In his popular book on trauma therapy, Van Der Kolk (2014) describes different therapies that work with these entities, such as internal family systems therapy (where part of the person and their defenses are objectified as separate entities), and psychomotor therapy (a specific technique using props for people in the patient's life). Gestalt therapy has been using similar techniques for decades. I have argued throughout this book that if it is to be analyzed, the zero process has to be approached on its own terms. And, to the extent that aspects of the trauma are independent centers of perception and feeling and initiative, they should be addressed as such. This extent varies, and I think that the manner in which they are addressed should reflect this—not for anything else, but because this has proven to be the most clinically effective way to do things.

The most robust evidence of the above assertions comes from experience of those treating DID. There, treating the alters as independent entities and talking to them as such, asking them what they are doing, what they know, asking them for help in mapping out other alters, making contracts with the more dangerous ones, or trying to ask them why they try to harm the person's body, and many other actions all acknowledge the independence of these entities and their level of complexity. Not doing this generally is either ineffective or at times harmful. At the same time, these entities are not actually separate people, with the complexity of a person, and thus things work best if they are not treated as such, or at least if this is kept in mind as the therapy moves forward. The alter is built around one or a few attitudes and emotional reactions, thoughts, beliefs and perceptions, and has only one form and content to their transference (also unlike a real, full person, who has a complex web of transferences), and the therapist in the end uses the communications with the alter to get at what these may be, so that these zero process memories can be accessed and processed. Usually once the alter has been accessed and brought into co-consciousness with other parts of the person, this processing takes place. In making these comments I leave out much of DID therapy related to the tactical aspects of learning about the existence of the alters, mapping them out, accessing them and working with them through hypnosis or other means, etc. I merely want to establish that accessing these zero process structures in the manner of their existence, if I could put it in such terms, is what aids the unraveling of the blocks to the natural automatic processing of the trauma.

The defense of splitting of the identity is a fascinating one, as it involves a combination of dynamics that build inner boundaries (repression) and outer ones (self/other differentiation). It captures the essence of the zero process as a set of experiences that stubbornly resist moving from something external to the mind to something internal to it. What I have found most helpful is working with the various entities created by this dynamic at a very concrete and specific level. This is different from inventing something general such as "your inner child" or "your damaged self" as a way to talk about a patient's experiences. The latter can be helpful, if such terms are suggested by the patient. They can at times shade into split off identities as true holders of parts of the trauma, but as general notions they are also prone to giving one a false sense of forward movement. There can, in my experience, be lots of emoting brought on by this type of work, but with little change. Many therapies address these kinds of more general entities, as do practitioners of dynamic psychotherapy. Some of the resistance to these techniques among psychoanalysts is because of these rather general, pop psychology aspects, which analysts rightly feel collapse many dynamics into an emotionally compelling but not very deep or accurate way of working. In contrast to this what I have in mind, as the product of splitting of the identity as a defense built on the original dissociation of major traumas, are a set of zero process memories, frozen into an identity that holds these memories, energized as a somewhat independent center of initiative, motivated by certain feelings and attitudes born from the trauma, and separated from the rest of the person by boundary-forming counterforce defenses.

I have found such entities are directly suggested by material that emerges as one explores a person's traumas, especially after one has gone a certain way into the trauma. I don't think it is very helpful to try and force the issue by inventing alters or identities that fit the bill. Much more transformational is when, as deeper memories of the trauma emerge the work itself, and the patient's manner of talking or feeling, suggest to the therapist or pateint the existence of an at least somewhat separate entity. This is the moment in which to talk about, and address, this entity as a separate being and see what happens. There may be a fear that such a comment will falsely create the entity by suggesting it to the patient, but to my mind, and in my experience, this does not happen if things are handled properly—by which I mean that the therapist's comments about the entity are treated like any other interpretation, as an intervention whose accuracy is judged by the patient's responses. And not just by the patient's yes or no, of course. The patient may find the idea intriguing and try and work with it, but not much will really emerge and the work will seem intellectual. Or—and this is usual, in my experience, when one is more on the mark—the patient may be very reluctant to talk of this experience as connected with an entity, and will need a little persuasion to at least give it a try and see what come to mind. And then something very powerful will emerge, that opens up areas of memory and feeling related to the trauma.

In my experience there is often a counter resistance to making these interpretations on the part of the therapist, a reluctance that I think is occasioned by the interpretation making real not just a specific identity split that belongs to the patient, but the whole idea and world of split off parts of people. Since every therapist will have at least some of these parts, as do we all, some portion of the reluctance to make these types of interpretations, especially when they are on the mark, will come from the therapist's own structure and defenses, just as all therapists have reluctance at times to interpret certain specific repressions of patients in relation to sexual and aggressive drive conflicts, because of the general human repression, including in the therapist, of such conflicts and fantasies. Analysis of identity splitting post-traumatic defenses in the therapist is helpful in mitigating this reluctance, and making them aware enough of them that they can spot their resistance and use it as a guide to spotting and interpreting this defense in others. The resistance never disappears, however, as these splits never do. I believe that, as with repression, some amount of the basic counterforce defense related to trauma and the zero process—identity splitting—as well as the other defenses that make up the central post-traumatic complex, are part of being human. Because of this, the dynamics of the central post-traumatic complex are important in various group and social phenomena.

What exactly do interventions related to identity splits look like? There is much literature on this, both in the treatment of full blown DID and in various techniques which use personification quite deliberately. In relation to the use of deliberate personification techniques, for instance in family systems therapy and many others, I have nothing to add, except to say that perhaps zero process theory can explain why and how and when these techniques work, and also their limitations. What I have tried to present are some thoughts on more specificity in techniques that work for entities related to splitting of the identity, the correct time to use them, and how to recognize this correct time. I would repeat that the timing is based on having gotten to concrete enough reactions in the trauma, having also traced their connection to the present, and using one's counter reactions, and counter resistances, to know when to interpret, and using the patient's reactions, as usual, to gauge the correctness of the interpretation and what to do next.

As an example, when discussing a patient's inability to stop moving, which she had had all her life, and having done a lot of work on a very early trauma of being hospitalized, left alone, and immobilized, which included the patient talking of having a feeling of often being separate from her body and dragging her somewhat inert body along, not being aware of its tiredness, or thirst, I made a comment. I said, "I wonder what the you that can't stop moving would say about the idea of stopping moving?" The patient talked in a somewhat intellectual manner about the need to move and its connection to the being restrained. "Maybe just ask her," I suggested. This comment was based on our having already talked extensively about the trauma, our making connections to present day reactions, and the patient herself introducing the feeling of dragging a body of a young girl around with her—which was her own body. The patient hesitated, and was silent, but something was clearly pushing to come out. It finally came out: "she would unravel … . If she stopped moving, she would unravel," she said, with intense emotion, starting to cry. This opened up many things: talk of what it felt like in the hospital, and specific experiences of being tied up. The little girl was tied up all night, night after night. Running around negated this, and put the trauma in the future. But to keep it in the future, she could not stop moving, both physically and in her mind. Importantly, there was a sense of this other reality, in the form of this other identity, coming into the session in a very immediate fashion. We were able to talk to this and other parts of the little girl, which all seemed related but also differentiated from each other as each was wrapped around different especially traumatic aspects of the hospitalization.

I don't think there is one way to do this type of work. It is more important to understand the dynamics of splitting of the identity, and understand and have experienced the concrete clinical issues around resistance and countertransference of resistance related to this type of split. The other point I would like to get across is that the work is really not different from any other interpretation of the unconscious and of defense, except for the form, of asking if the identities have anything to add. Sometimes you can talk directly to them, sometimes as you ask, the patient will tell you what they are saying or feeling or doing. The main thing is to be open minded in listening to what happens, and then use this as a guide as one tries to help the process of exploration, evocation, and integration. In my experience what works is to go about the analysis with split off identities in a natural way, following them into the depths of the trauma if they lead you there, or letting them say a few words and returning to them later if that is where the patient's associations go.

In order to illustrate some of what I have said about analyzing the zero process and zero process defenses I will close this section, and this chapter, with some clinical material from the patient who began this book: Cordelia. The sessions come a few years after the ones I detailed earlier. At this point we had talked about ending and had set a date. The end date was about seven months ahead of the sessions below. I had thought of giving a good deal of time for the termination phase, as I expected a lot that would need to be worked through in relation to final endings. I was explicit with her about my thinking, and asked her for her thoughts when I brought up the possibility of ending. Cordelia was doing much better—for instance in being able to stand up for herself. But what really convinced me that we may be able to terminate and work through the transference issues related to loss was that she was doing a lot of the work, and producing a lot of the insights, by herself. She seemed able to work at two levels much more consistently—both having reactions and resistances related to her transference and past dynamics, and at the same time having ideas into what these meant which were not an intellectual overlay, but seemed to be genuine flashes of true insight. As usual, I am frustrated at only being able to present, because of considerations of space, a few snippets from my quite copious notes from these session. The clinicians who are reading this will be able to understand just what a small bit of what actually happened is presented here. I will supplement my extracts from the notes with comments, in square bracket.

A few months after we had decided on the date to end, the coronavirus struck. We began seeing each other via video. Many of my patients, either to start out with or as time progressed, were treated via either phone or other audio connections, as this often seemed to work best, with no lag. But I had a feeling Cordelia would need to keep seeing my face at this time. I discussed this with her, and she was clear, with no hesitation, that this was what she would prefer. At one point during the time of the sessions described below, I asked her again, and she said she preferred video because "you are closer to me, on the screen, than in person." As one might imagine, this had many meanings, and hid many feelings about the changes in our therapy, as well as about the ending.

Here are selections from my session notes: she is permeated by a negative feeling towards her present employer. [she has been thinking of retiring in a year or two. She is working full time remotely.] She wonders if it's like her tendency to move on from men and feel they are bad for her or that there's something damaging about being with them and also with the employer. She then says a little sheepishly that she had a "hysterical fit" at two meetings. It started with laughing—a full throated laughter. "I felt like I hadn't laughed like that so fully in a very long time." At the end this evolved into crying, also full throated. She says that they both seemed—she then searches for a word that could describe it, and settles on "honest." She describes the first situation, on a zoom call with a number of people in a group she's in. Somebody did something, moved in a funny way, and she started laughing but then found she couldn't stop and started to move off the screen and then to her surprise it turned into crying. "Very deep crying." She goes into a bit more description of the two situations. She talks about how she wants to leave her employer in order to take up a new position, and how she has it set up in her mind so the place that she's going seems so ideal. [I noticed that she has been able in relation to these changing and very strong feelings about her present employer, with whom she has been with for over a decade, to both have these feelings, and in quite a clear eyed way to see that they are related to something else.] In relation to what she's saying I note how excited she was when she heard her stepmother was coming [after her mother's death]. I wonder out loud if she had developed a fantasy of the ideal perfect mother, whom she then expected her stepmother to be. She says her stepmother acted more like a sister, an envious older sister: cold, harsh. This replaced her mother. She looked forward to the new mother. She was very excited, and pictured her as the perfect mother. She thinks that it somehow has to do with her aggression as well, she says. [I think as she says this that she is again demonstrating an easy ability to move back-and-forth between experiencing and these sorts of deeper insights.] I mention the fear of people, and of dogs. She talks about her dream of the murderous farmer—her first dream in therapy. She talks about her two mothers. And I bring out how her biological mother [I say the name] was warmer, and then she left and maybe the patient was caught. She felt she had to leave her after she died, in order not to be dead. [I am at this point thinking of the moment when her father had said that her mother was not coming back. Cordelia had felt a black thing enter through her belly, and go into her. At this point it strikes me that the black cloud was both death and her own aggression, but also how terrifying it would have been to feel pulled towards this death.] The patient wonders about her anger and turning it inwards against herself. She then talks of how petty and aggressive and envious she can get with coworkers and the people she is supposed to manage. She says she reminds herself of her stepmother. [again I get the feeling she is on a roll. She does not seem to be beating herself up, just observing.] I say that this was another internalization, taking place in adolescence, as she tried to break away from her stepmother.

"But I didn't get enough from her!"

"Or from [her mother—we are saying the names]." She talks of still wanting to get the mothering from her different mothers. "So maybe it's something that stays with me—it's like I go back and forth between one mother and the other. And I hope when I go to the new situation all the frustrations won't be there, but of course I take myself to the new situation, so it's still the same me." She describes how when she left her marriage she was the one who left, but then became desperate as if she had been the one who had been abandoned. "It's like I leave but I am also left."

"That happened to you not just when your mother left when she died, but also in adolescence in a way. [your stepmother] had not been the mother you wanted so you leave but she has already left; she's not around." We talk about this some more and it is clearly something that's affecting her. As it's time to end and I say so. She says that she has developed a rash just then. Cordelia shows me her right forearm, holding it up to the video. It has a number of red raised spots on it. I ask her if it just started, and she says yes it started just now. We are already at the end, so we don't have time to analyze it. She seems quite struck by what has happened, as am I.

Next session, two days later [we see each other two sessions per week]: She says that she has "bug bite" like lesions. They are raised red areas smaller than a small coin. She has them on both forearms. She says that the gloomy mood and negativity that she was feeling just before and during the last session disappeared as these lesions appeared. She says of the spots, "I don't mind them so much – they're better than the feelings." She seems to mean this, and to be in quite a good mood but also to be sincerely reporting how bad the feelings were and how much nicer it is just to have the rash. She says she had been feeling very sorry for herself, very negative, and very victimized. "I don't like feeling that way, but it just comes over me. I had a couple of dreams over the last few days."

Dream—she is back in the home environment of her first long-term boyfriend. "It was a wonderful home, of wealth, of progressive ideas." She goes on to describe how different it was from her more conservative and more working class home. She says in the dream she was wondering if she would get together with him but then realized there was another woman there. She realizes they would not get together. She sees them (he and the woman) taking a bath in the sink. It seems somehow perfectly normal. She realizes in the end that she doesn't mind that she can't get together with him. She has her true love here with her present husband and does not need anyone else. [end]

In thinking of the dream she notes that the sink reminds her that her mother would bathe both her, and after her brother was born her and her brother, in the kitchen sink. She has pictures of this. She laughs in a playful way as she remembers this. [I am thinking that with this boy-friend too, it was 4 years that they were together—as long as her mother and her.] She says about the dream that she was at first jealous of this other woman but then somehow came around to feeling much better, and to appreciating what she has in the present. She thinks that must be what the dream is about. She would always yearn for the people and things that she had decided to leave, but in the dream she is appreciating what she has in the present instead of this yearning. Cordelia then recounts another dream.

Dream—She is with her grandmother all night long in her grandmother's house. It's full of all sorts of special objects and her grandmother is explaining each of them. She is explaining what they are. Cordelia is able to take any of them. It seems like a kind of dowery that her grandmother is giving her. [end]

Cordelia says the dream seemed full of abundance and possibility. She realizes that there was a lot of the colour green in both of the dreams. This leads me to wonder about a connection to childbirth. I note that her brother's birth must have been the first time that she felt envy and jealousy in a very big way. Perhaps the two dreams show us the connections between this, her anger at her mother and jealousy around her brother's birth (and her sister's after this), and perhaps the way this got entwined with the next major time her mother left her, which was when she died. And this was around the time when she was feeling jealous of her mother in relation to her father as well, so these things all got mixed up together. This might be shown especially in the second dream with all these beautiful things which were her dowry for marriage. And then the green which related to having children may connect her brother's birth, her sister's birth, her envy, and her own wishes regarding having children. We talk of this, and I make comments about what she was talking about, about the aggression, and then about turning it against herself. There is something of that in the physical complaints that have dogged her ever since childhood and adolescence, which took specific form in early adulthood, but which already had to do with her stomach in her childhood when she would get bad stomach aches. We talk of her longing towards mothers, and her anger at them and her wish to identify with them and then the fear of this—but she could never be finished with the two of them, because she had never gotten enough from them, so she clung to them even as she tried to separate. We discuss something of the trauma living in her future, so that she was trying to solve it, by finding the perfect mother, but she was scared to settle down, because this would lead to the trauma no longer being in the future. [We have discussed this before, but this time it seems more real, and she seems to resonate with it. What is especially real is how by this temporal shift, she was robbed of a realistic future of staying with a person and having children, which she wanted.] So she ran. She left before she was traumatically left, as she had said, and so she lived at the point where she was still struggling, where she could not remember perhaps the full throated honest laughter that she had shared with her mother, because if she started doing that, she would also remember the terrible loss, and so she avoided the full throated crying for what she had lost. She seems to connect to this discussion at a deep emotional level. It was something, the laughing/crying, that happened after the session with me, she says. She was embarrassed by what happened but not disturbed or shattered. In fact, she smiles as she talks of what happened, and seems to have gotten relief from it.

In the next session Cordelia recounts an incident in detail, in which a familiar sequence played out, where she jumped to aid someone with a physical ailment, but then panicked that her intervention may have hurt them. In relation to her feeling as if she has caused harm to people she's trying to save I wonder about her theories regarding her mother's death. Did she perhaps think that her anger had caused her death or played a part in it? She says that what comes to mind is the feeling of being abandoned—of being so alone. She goes on to talk about her dad saying her mother was not coming back. I ask her to say some more about that. She says that perhaps another kid would've thought that maybe her mother would come back at some other date. I say that might've been different for her because there was a build up where her mother had been so ill in hospital. She says that's very true. "I knew it was over. That she was not coming back," she says in an eerily sad voice. We talk some more about this. About the darkness of death going inside her as she realized this. About her identification with her mother, and her having to then pull away. This connects with her having talked about feeling kind of identified with the person she was trying to help the day before, as if she and they were one.

Cordelia goes on to talk about the way she has certain "hysterical" reactions with people that gives them a bad impression and leads them to react to her in a negative way. "These hysterical reactions have been happening quite a bit lately. I want to be over that." I point out that she is having some very strong reactions including what she called hysterical reactions of laughing and crying. In that case she found the reactions somewhat releasing and relieving. I say I think that stuff is starting to bubble up because of the ending and because of our work at the moment. She talks about the past living with her and about trying to stave off the death. I say that perhaps the death lives in her future. She is always working to avoid it. Perhaps as we have looked in more detail at what happened at that moment when her father told her that her mother was not coming home, we can see that she tries to live at the time just before that, when she could still save her mother. We now know that her panic and hysteria might be because she knows what's coming. It's completely real because it was real. That traumatic moment when her father told her and then she knew that her mother was never coming back is what looms in her future, and she has spent so much of her present trying to make that not happen, and avoid certain things in the future because this "future memory" crowded them out. [This temporal shifting, along with the identity split related to her aggression and abandonment illustrated just below, made up Cordelia's central post-traumatic complex.]

At the next session, Cordelia goes to remembering the time in early adulthood when she got quite sick with what seem to have been psychologically caused symptoms. She went home wanting her stepmother to take care of her, but neither she nor her father showed much interest.

"I probably wondered when my mother died who was going to take care of me. Who was going to be concerned about me?" [at this point I get a very strong feeling, and an image, of her mother and her concern for the patient when she was a young girl, and a deep feeling of sadness about the loss of that.] "I was really surprised at the lack of concern. I did feel I was looking for it, and maybe I played a part. I don't know how much I helped create that situation." At this point she looks up and notices a bird through her window. [She is at home, connecting virtually with me.] "Those are the cardinals that were nesting in the rosebush last year. We watched the young ones and they finally took flight on July first. [It's now the beginning of June of the next year, 2020. The pandemic is raging.] I think those are the same birds and it's amazing to see the parents feeding them still. They don't have the colouration but they're almost as big as their parents. Maybe it's time for the young birds to be on their own." Cordelia talks about various plants in her garden and house and the animals around outside. "I get so much pleasure from keeping things alive" We talk about how that happens to the point where she can be quite intrusive in terms of other people.

"I think I'm taking care of them the way I want to be taken care of."

"And maybe the desperation and pushiness, it's because that part of you that is still back there is desperate for caring, also desperate to keep your mother alive, both those things. The people whom you are trying to help may not see it is such an emergency situation and may find your anxiety and pushiness irritating. But if you think about it in terms of yourself, your mother is dying and nothing has helped so you're desperate, and at the same time because your mother is dead you are desperate to get the caring that you used to get from her and dealing with the bereft feeling that you will never get that again."

In the rest of the session we take up these issues in relation to the therapy. "I'm waiting less for things," she says, and I note perhaps she has gotten better because now the waiting for the perfect mother to appear is lived out in here. Maybe the symptoms have returned and some of the progress has reversed as we talk of the ending here, because previously she may have had a feeling that it would not end here. She says that it's true. She thought there would be something she would get from here. "I feel I want something from here. And I don't really feel ready for it to end." "Can you picture being ready?" "No, not really." "Maybe what you live out with me is ending too soon, as with your mother, before you got all you needed from her. There is never a good time to end here, because it was not a good time to end with your mother."

In the next session Cordelia talks of other instances in the present where people did not respond to her as she expected, and she reacted very strongly. "The lack of response from others leads me to spiral away from myself." We look at how she internalizes her anger at other people. She feels she did not get enough from her mother – "and from the therapy", I add. We discuss the transference implications of this.

In the session after this one, Cordelia says that she is feeling overall better, but still a bit up and down. "I've been feeling better ever since I got the hives." She details how the hives have moved to her legs—still not very severe. She notes how she has often gotten different physical symptoms and says she thinks its related to her aggression. [She had developed pains and contracture on her right side, related to anger at, and a wish to hit, her husband—see the section "Triggers, Repetitions, and Conversion Symptoms" in chapter one.] She brings up in relation to this the very first dream she had while in therapy, of the psychopath who was killing the farmers and piling them up under a bridge. She talks about the details of this dream. She says that when she saw the killer she was frozen. There was a dark brown man standing off to the side watching. [I am brown skinned.] Her friend was with her. The psychopath turned to look at her and this is when she felt frozen. Her friend was telling her that they had to run but she couldn't. The dead men are like farmers with bibs that the farmers wear—bib overalls. One of them starts to stir, showing he's not dead yet, and the psychopath takes a shovel and smashes him over the head to kill him. As we talk about her anger being embodied in the psychopath, the patient says, "but psychopaths aren't really curable, are they? So I wonder how I would be able to get over this rage." I say it's not really a person but an embodiment of a specific feeling from a specific time. It's like the alters in DID. They have only a few feelings or actions which they repeat endlessly, suggesting their derivation from a frozen piece or pieces of traumatic experiences. I would think this psychopath is like that, some piece of her experience frozen and embodied sometimes in a psychopath in her dream, sometimes in the black dog who will attack her. Are these all an embodiment of the rage from the trauma of the loss of her mother frozen in time rather than capable of being modified and growing up with her? I say that her anger and the trauma of her mother's death seem to be almost fused together. She listens very intently, nodding thoughtfully but not saying anything. I bring up how she had the experience of the black cloud entering through her stomach when her dad told her about her mother's death. And the dream of the black dog jumping at her stomach. I say that my feeling is that this black cloud represented both death and her anger fused together and that I think this is different even then feeling that her mother's death was caused by her anger. I say that I think it is an actual fusion in which the two things are one in a very concrete way.

In the next session, Cordelia starts by talking of her sense of not being secure. What does this mean? People see her as self-confident, she says, but – the little girl that is also there is different. She says she abandons herself as she abandons others. Then is resentful of others and has "seething anger," as she calls it. She begins to wonder what the word "seething" really means. "Is it bubbling? ... It's painful; it creates a kind of aloneness. But I do it to myself. I go into myself and I'm bubbling." This is the seething anger. I interpret that this might have been first felt at her sibling's birth, first one and then the other. These were the other times that she felt excluded or lost her mother. "It's an age when there is so much dependence on the mother" Cordelia says. She pictures herself all by herself, seething. I bring up how this can also be a positive experience of independence, and that it throws you back on yourself and fosters your differentiation from your mother. But, with her mother's death, this positive aspect of what happened earlier was partly lost. "I never got a chance to repair that. I transferred it to my grandmother, who was warm and motherly, but I cried very deeply every time I had to leave her house at the end of the weekend to go back to my parent's place and my stepmother. My stepmother took it personally as an affront to her. But it really was something else."

"Your grandmother could help you and soothe you to some extent, but we can see that somehow the loss in its traumatic aspect was withdrawn from change. You relived it every time."

At the next session, Cordelia exclaims that she loves the summer. We have talked of this before, how in the middle of winter she always wants to, and often does, go down south. She talks of how in the summer, there's the birds, the animals. "It's bleak in winter. I feel I just curl up" "I wonder if in winter you go inside yourself, and it can be bleak." "I want to convert my inside to have summer." We talk about this whole issue of warmth and how she needs the warmth from outside, because she still needs her mother. When her mother died it was winter in her mind, she says. We implicitly are connecting this to our talk previously about never having been able to fully take in and internalize the warmth and love of her mother.

She says that she had "quite a dream" – a dead body. The body of a young boy who had very thick hair, like a girl. She looked out the window and saw animals. A brown and white owl sat beside each other on a branch, which was magical. Then a wolf and rabbit were there. The wolf grabbed the rabbit, and she went out trying to save it, opening the back door. "I couldn't get there in time and the wolf caught the rabbit and ran off with it. I was upset at first, but then I was OK with it. It seemed like the way nature works. The wolf had to eat too." She goes from this to talking about the child again. She had guilt for it but no idea or information on how it all came about. She had to hide the body and there was desperation on her side about how to do this, about being found out, and about not knowing why she was guilty or what she had done or how the body had come to be there.

Many things come out from this dream. Cordelia notes that the situation with the child's body was nightmarish. I point out that she had guilt but no information and this may be a representation of the time after her mother's death. People have not told her about what had happened. She had not gone to the funeral and her dad did not talk about her mother after her death very much at all, I say. So maybe this is a representation of the bleak period after her death, I continue, along with the guilt that she felt. She talks of having to cut off the hair of the dead boy. Like she would be cutting off his power. It makes her think of Jungian ideas, about her feeling her animus, which is her male part, was cut off around the age of 12. I connect this perhaps with her start of menstruation and definitive body and gender choice, while before this things were more fluid. She notes that it was around the age that her father married her stepmother. I note that this may then have been the cutting off of her Oedipal wishes. She said she had to bury the body six feet down and it felt impossible that she would be ever be able to dig that deep, but somehow she had to do it anyway and she set herself to the task. [In the sessions after this, it becomes clear through her associations that the dead body is her from childhood, related to a part of her that carries the trauma and holds onto death and a connection with her dead mother. She previously had dreamt of dead bodies, that she had to hide or found and realized that she had killed them. These were a combination of her mother and the split identity that was still fused with her.]

We end up talking about how the two owls might be her and I, me as the brown one. She adds to this that the owls were watching what was happening the way we watch and talk about her life and things in it. "Somehow the scene seemed OK. I was OK with what was taking place. I didn't have to save the rabbit." I say that this may be the future that she wishes for—when she doesn't have to save every vulnerable thing. She looks out into her future, but in the house is the dead body and the guilt and the gender and oedipal issues. This is her bleak inside, and she is looking outside, to the future that she hopes for. "I want to have the sunshine and warmth inside as well. It's happening now, to some extent."

A few weeks after the interactions above, Cordelia starts the session talking again about how she likes the warm weather, which leads us to talk of her mother's death. When I mention the darkness that went inside her she says, "it was emptiness that went inside me. I was empty after that." She then ends up talking of her anger about the ending of the therapy, although she doesn't sound very angry as she says it. I point this out to her, and she says that sometimes she is naive, like a little child. I ask her about this different part of her. "It's like a naive little child." "Is it also angry?" "No. I feel if I let it come out, I just start to cry. And it feels like the crying just won't stop." [I have noted in the section "Some Applications" in chapter two, that Volkan (2014) described perennial mourning in patients for whom the mourning is never over, and the lost person is ever present. Cordelia's case demonstrates the dynamic of perennial mourning as connected to splitting of the identity with one identity containing the sadness and loss. In such cases, as long as the alter is not integrated with the rest of the personality, the mourning will never be over. One can be easily fooled as a therapist into believing that the patient just needs to feel the sadness more and emote more for a therapeutic result—but this is not the case. Cordelia cried, from the start of the therapy, easily and often about her mother's death. But there was no change that came from these emotional expressions.]

"But the little child has no anger?" I asked.

"No."

"But it did seem like the psychopath in your dreams and other killers—they are also a part of you."

"That's different. That feels like a teenager. A teenage boy, 14 maybe. He's angry."

"And does he have something to tell us?"

"Fuck Off!" Cordelia says, in a more forceful voice than is usual for her, even when angry. She seems to startle herself somewhat, and laughs. She is taking a sip of her tea as she says this. As far as I can see from the video, the exclamation takes her by surprise, startling her, and some of the tea spills. "I spilled some tea on myself," she says.

"Anything else?"

Cordelia seems to be accessing her mind, as she has an inward look, and then says, "no, only that. 'Fuck Off!' That's all he has to say. He doesn't seem to have many words to describe what he went through. Just 'Fuck Off! Fuck Off!' Cordelia laughs again as she says this. I notice that the voice sounds different, when Cordelia says, "Fuck Off!"

During the next session, we talk about how Cordelia often expresses herself through physical symptoms, and I comment that this is especially common in younger children. She describes again the crying little girl and how she feels it through her body. Not really pain as such, but something not right throughout her body. Then Cordelia again mentions the angry teenage boy, and says that she thinks that he is related to how difficult her stepmother was. She has mentioned some of the incidents she now proceeds to describe, the details of which I will not describe for reasons of confidentiality, but this time around they are much more real, and the feelings not just stronger but more integrated one with the other. She notes that this split between the good mother and the bad mother may have been fostered because her grandmother was so much like a good mother. "I could just curl up with her. She always made my favourite foods. At the end of the weekend I had to go back to my home and my stepmother." This is a point she has made and described previously, including how she would cry each Sunday when she had to go back. But with this too, something is different, in how real and immediate the description feels. I think at the time that it is something about having evoked the part of her, the teenage boy. It is not as uncanny as a completely separate alter talking, but in a more subtle but quite powerful manner it is like a different voice is now getting its chance to tell the story.

Cordelia talks about the ways in which her stepmother had curtailed her moves towards independence. "I guess they are kind of small things, but for me they were big." In fact they seemed quite big to me as well, when she described them in telling detail. Even her reasonable moves towards independence were harshly curtailed and attacked by her stepmother. Now she relived the fight for independence and separation of adolescence, and over the next number of sessions this got connected back to her anger at her mother for getting sick and dying. We saw how this had been split off, and this split off aspect rekindled in the normative regression to early childhood during early adolescence. This regression was, as usual, quite deep, and it revived her early trauma, its zero process memories, and the split identities and split mother imagos built around these memories. This is normative, and can be growth promoting as the trauma is acted out in the present and reworked in various ways. Cordelia's situation more hindered than helped her. Her aggression, which is usually accessed through the adolescent regression, was definitively locked up in the young adolescent boy, and was not as available for the final separation from childhood and childhood figures. The outcome of childhood traumas that we see in adults is always, and usually in quite decisive ways, refracted through the adolescent process. It is only once the particularities of this adolescent refraction are brought to light and worked through that deeper change of repetitions and symptoms related to early traumas takes place.

During the session described, it feels like an important piece of Cordelia's history is making a direct appearance. I point out to her that the split between her stepmother and maternal grandmother probably was a hiding place for an original set of split feelings towards her biological mother. I say that there were many causes for her anger, including the birth of her siblings, her mother's abandonment of her through her difficult illness, and then the final abandonment of her mother's death. I say even the best mother will at times make her child angry and even be hated by them because of the frustrations that they impose, but that this is not usually a problem. In fact the anger powers separation and a firming up of the self. But her mother's death had frozen a split between

these feelings, normal for such a young age. Then this split was con-
solidated throughout her childhood and adolescence by what she described with her grandmother and stepmother. Often adolescence is a
second chance to rework traumas from the past. Rather than being reworked, the split between the good mother Cordelia mourned (the crying
child) and the bad mother she hated (the "fuck off!" child and then
adolescent) was reinforced by the family situation and her stepmother's
treatment of her. A number of these things had been said before and
some, such as her reactions to the birth of her two siblings, had been
analyzed quite often and from many angles. But at this point it seemed to
me that it was time for a more integrating narrative reconstruction of the
origin and fate of Cordelia's split mother and split identity.

Our accessing of Cordelia's split identities and my reconstruction related to them seemed to help the process along, as over the next number
of sessions more material emerged relating to Cordelia's adolescence and
certain difficulties in the development of her identity. She realized that
she had always felt incomplete without a man, but that she usually left
these men, a number of them at around the four year mark in their relationship, but then felt that they had abandoned her. While there were
oedipal elements in these actions, they were also regressively related to
her complex feelings of love and anger towards her mother, and her
difficulties in forging a fully separate identity from her. Cordelia at this
point has a dream with a dangerous man and teenage boy, with the boy
coming to join her, leaving the man. This she feels is a part of her coming
back to her from the man.

In the next session, in talking about some very different opinions and
views of the world of her stepmother as compared to her own, Cordelia
describes how a friend of hers had said, in relation to this, "she's not your
biological mother." "I know that's true, intellectually," Cordelia says,
"but it came to me like a kind of shock. It's like it penetrated deeper this
time. I feel like I'm separating from [she says the name of her stepmother.]" [I'm thinking to myself, now that she has reclaimed the "Fuck
Off!" teenager, and he is starting to be more integrated with her, she is
able to use that energy to separate.] Cordelia says that she can feel and
see her biological mother more now. "She is more alive and real to me
now. Which is funny, that now I feel I accept her death more fully. But
she is more alive to me."

"It seems contradictory only on the surface. At a deeper level it makes
sense. Your mother existed before only as a dying mother, or one who
had just died. She was frozen in time. Now that she is becoming un-
frozen, and you accept her death more, she can exist as more of a whole
and alive person inside of you."

"I feel like I'm getting my family back. [My stepmother] always criti-
cized my grandmother. She tried to suppress the sense of family." There

was a very intense feeling in this, which I could feel very well even over the video. The feeling was one of becoming whole. It wasn't one of being furious at her stepmother. These things had been described by Cordelia previously, often with anger. Now there was firmness, which led to more of a feeling of separateness, both from her stepmother and from her mother. Cordelia could see her stepmother not as the evil stepmother of fairy tales, but as a limited and insecure woman. She had never actually been able to poison Cordelia's relationship with her maternal grandmother or her biological mother, but Cordelia had still remained stuck as the upset teenager in relation to her. Now that she had reclaimed the aggression tied up in the "Fuck Off" teenager, she could sublimate it and use it, to move on from her stepmother and, at the deepest level, to separate herself from her dying mother. This did not happen all at once. But the more Cordelia could separate from her dying mother, and let her die, without feeling herself pulled into death with her, the more her mother came alive inside her. "I am filled with the presence of her," she said.

In the following sessions, Cordelia was more and more connected to a complex, whole, inner mother representation. What helped this was also work on another split identity, of the little girl who had experienced the time after her mother's death, which Cordelia had tried to keep at a distance. This identity contained the core of the early trauma and the zero process drive that came from it, and deep structural changes came from Cordelia's reconciling with her, against strong resistance and requiring working through of a good deal of guilt about having abandoned the little traumatized girl—she was one part of all the dead people Cordelia kept finding behind walls and in other places in her dreams, not knowing where they came from or how she came into possession of their bodies. In relation to the split identities, I want to stress again the need for directive interventions at times. It was in evidence in bringing up the teenage identity, but sometimes I find an explicit statement, something like what is done in working with DID, is helpful. For instance, in relation to the little girl identity I said to Cordelia, "If the young girl that is from the time we are talking about has anything to say, maybe she can say it." If timed correctly this type of intervention has enormous power. It is also open to abuse leading to a false covering over of other issues by talking to various inner entities. This is why I have tried to give at least a few more detailed examples, to show how this type of intervention is best when one has already done lots of preliminary work, and the existence of the identity split is quite obvious, as it has emerged organically from analytic work, and becomes accessible.

In this last excerpt from Cordelia's therapy, I have painted a portrait of how analyzing the zero process defenses of temporal shifting and splitting of the identity frees up the zero process, and all that it has become entangled with. In Cordelia's case, her aggression had become fused with the death of her mother, and frozen in a moment in time. The zero process memories related to her mother's illness and death had become embedded in her emotional conflicts related to her siblings, in her sexual and gender conflicts, and in her Oedipal wishes and conflicts. Only by taking Cordelia's identities seriously as separate entities could the zero process memories that they were built upon, and stabilized by, be freed up. Once this was achieved, the actual living out of the memories so that they are finally laid to rest became possible. There was much working through and much struggle, but as the zero process memories were finally brought to light, they were at times integrated in a surprisingly automatic manner, as happens in bland traumas. This allowed the conflicts in which they had become embedded to be analyzed.

Summary

The field of trauma therapy is large and diverse. I have in this chapter described some ideas on technique which flow from zero process theory, and tried to situate these within this larger field. I can imagine that some of what I have said, about the need for active exploration of trauma, confrontation of avoidance defenses in both patient and therapist, and direct engagement with separate identities built around zero process memories, may be met with skepticism by some psychoanalysts and psychodynamic therapists. I hope that by making my points about therapeutic interventions in the context of an explication of the nature of trauma, post-traumatic functioning, and post-traumatic dynamics, they can be seen as reasonable and helpful steps in the analysis of trauma.

Conclusion

In the first section of chapter two ("Traumatic Memories and the Construction of Reality") I described a patient of William Niederland's (1965) who was considered schizophrenic because he wore his coat even in the hottest summer weather. It turned out he had almost frozen to death before his first year. His behaviour, shivering in Niederland's office with a winter coat on, is a dramatic demonstration of the nature of zero process memory, which behaves like a present experience and thus sets up an alternate second reality. It also sets up an alternate second future. Niederland's freezing patient was not actually frozen almost to death in the present. He was shivering and had his coat on, trying to keep warm. The height of his trauma, almost frozen to death and then almost dying of pneumonia in the hospital, lay in his future, and he was hard at work trying to fend it off with shivering and winter coats. In this we have a clear demonstration of the structure of the central post-traumatic complex.

I concluded the last chapter with some excerpts demonstrating the dynamics and structures that developed in the aftermath of the traumas suffered by my patient Cordelia. I began the first chapter of this book by describing the worst of these traumas: hearing of the death of her mother when she was four. As we journeyed from the description of Cordelia's trauma, and those of Peggy and Joyce, to the details of their analyses, I attempted to map out some of the landscape of trauma. My aim in this book has been to use psychoanalytic investigational methods to draw a more accurate map of the land of trauma. I wanted to go deep in relation to key details, for instance about the nature of memory functioning during and after trauma, and of post-traumatic defenses and psychodynamics. My hope was that with this more accurate map in hand, we would be able to approach other facets of trauma, and mental dynamics more generally, and garner new insights. I will conclude by mentioning a few of the conceptual landmarks touched on in this work, in terms of further research that could be undertaken in relation to them.

Trauma was described as a situation that overwhelms the mind, leading to the breakdown of the first-order construction of the present moment. This unconstructed present is the zero process. We can see its characteristics in Niederland's patient. His coldness is unconnected with other memories or knowledge related to the incident, and it imposes itself on him as a present experience and future fear. In relation to the consequences of this breakdown of construction we could ask, what about when the tools to construct reality don't yet exist, or are in a rudimentary state—in other words, in early infancy? This leads to what I call the **developmental zero process** (see glossary), which follows us all our lives as a background second reality. And this also leads to a broader topic: the connection of trauma and development. Much has been written about this, but I would hope that armed with a clearer conceptual understanding of the nature of post-traumatic mental functioning, we could add to this discussion, for instance in relation to the sublimation of trauma into people's passions, and the interweaving of the developmental zero process, the zero process proper, and ego and emotional development.

I have drawn a rather sharp distinction between the zero process as a product of the breakdown of reality construction, and other forms of mental functioning. But what about boundary situations of extreme strain and chronic impingements that do not fully rise to the level of severe trauma? In this book, I have mainly opted for a deeper investigation into the zero process proper. But from the vantage point gained from these investigations, a different conceptualization of strain and stress and developmental interferences of various sorts comes into view. An investigation of this area too, I plan to undertake in my next book.

I described briefly the manner in which the zero process serves as the core of introjects and alters. It is what makes them independent centers of initiative, and gives them many of their other qualities, such as the tendency to repeat the same reactions over and over. An enhanced understanding of the developmental and dynamic aspects of introjects can be applied to the structure that partially absorbs and influences them: the superego. I think that zero process theory could not just lead to further ideas about the superego, but could revolutionize our view of the internal object world more generally, as we may come to see that it actually consists of two worlds: one, related to the zero process, that is much more external to the mind than, and has quite different properties from, the other.

We have seen how understanding the nature of the zero process allows a clearer view of the dynamics of intergenerational transmission of trauma, as the non-traumatized person constructs for themselves, from zero process bits and pieces, the trauma of the traumatized person, and feels it as their own. This dynamic also explains, I believe, the intergenerational transmission of our quintessential zero process structure, the superego, including its ideals, and has very wide application in relation to the transmission of ethnic and cultural ideals, ideologies, and identities, and thus socio-historical processes. This is an area of active investigation among analysts, to which zero process theory can make important additions. Further afield, but not as much further as it may at first appear, is the question of the evolutionary origins of the human mind, and here too an understanding of the zero process aspects of internal objects, the superego, and intergenerational transmission will be of help, I believe, in constructing an evolutionary psychoanalysis.

As I bid the reader goodbye, I would like to stress that while the concepts and theories in this book may have been presented in a manner that suggests a complete system, they are only the first steps in developing what I hope is a more extensive and more accurate theory. What I have presented are some outlines of a rough map of the area of the mind that comes into existence after trauma. As noted in the introduction, the first explorers in the land of trauma mistook it for other places in the mind, such as the deeper emotional mind of primal fantasies and powerful emotional conflicts. I have suggested instead that the mind is simply a much bigger place than was originally imagined, and than many people may imagine still. There is no reason to throw out or diminish the importance of Freud's great discoveries, or of more recent work on early neglect and other major interferences in development, in order to make room for trauma. Nor do we need to reduce trauma to one of these things, such as emotional conflicts or developmental interferences. Our minds contain multitudes. One of the guiding ideas in this book is that by more clearly understanding what trauma is not, we will more deeply understand what it is. I hope I have provided the reader with a better map of this terrain, including the areas still in need of further voyages of exploration and discovery.

Glossary

Attentional Defense A form of defense, usually directed against un-pleasant realities (internal or external) which uses shifting of atten-tion as its basis, and other higher level ego capacities such as thinking and suppression as supplements. Denial is the classic attentional defense, but there are others such as rationalization and some forms of internalizing and externalizing defenses (see Fernando, 2009, for elaboration on these).

Bland Trauma In this form of trauma, the traumatic process of ego shutdown takes place, leaving unprocessed zero process memories, but the push to relive and process these memories belatedly is able to proceed unhindered and go to completion. Bland trauma is im-portant practically and theoretically, in showing us in clear terms how recovery can happen after trauma, leading us to ask why it doesn't in so many cases, and showing us what we need to do therapeutically to heal trauma.

Central Post-Traumatic Complex This term designates a set of zero process defenses that are used to keep zero process memories from playing out fully in the present. The main defenses are splitting of the identity and temporal shifting. Through these defenses, the zero process drive and zero process memories are contained within certain identities and kept at a distance, in the person's future. The central post-traumatic complex leads to situation that can be mistaken for repetition, but that involves living at points just before the full shattering effects of the trauma were felt — these effects having been relegated to the future and to other identities. Through the magic of the zero process and zero process defenses, the project of changing the past can be felt as possible. But the dictates of reality mean that it can never become actual. The person must remain in the constant balance of living at the point just before the trauma happened. Because the central post-traumatic com-plex bars the automatic reliving/healing/integrative post-traumatic processes from taking place, its analysis is one key to trauma therapy.

Compound Defense This type of defense is composed of two or more basic processes, such as higher level ego capacities like thinking and a counterforce (obsessional defenses), or dissociation and a counterforce (splitting of the identity), which act in concert and are tightly bound together. In the case of defenses acting together that are not compounded, once can generally analyze each defense separately. The inability to do this indicates that the defenses are more tightly bound into a compound defense.

Contrast Defense In this type of defense the person avoids realities that contrast too much with a distressing reality that they are trying to avoid, because of the tendency of the contrasting reality to evoke the distressing one. A situation that contrasts too strongly with a trauma upsets the balance of the **central post-traumatic complex** by evoking the feeling that the trauma is now over (rather than the trauma still being about to happen in the future), and that it's now time to process it.

Counterforce Defense A form of defense directed usually against a drive derivative or strong affect related to a zero process or id drive. This type of defense uses a powerful counterforce to push its objects out of awareness, and to keep them unconscious. Well functioning counterforce defenses form stable barriers. The counterforce itself is formed from partially neutralized aggressive drive energy. Partially neutralized aggression is used to set up other stable mental barriers, such as self/other boundaries, and the self/self boundaries of splitting of the identity.

Developmental Zero Process This term refers to memories from the first year of life, formed before such capacities as symbolization and higher level integrative capacities have developed. Thus these memories are not constructed enough to become part of the person's past, do not acquire narrative structure, and survive as a background canvas upon which the present reality that follows is painted. By the latter part of the first year as the ego develops the developmental zero process gives way to more regular memories that are situated in the person's past, and as the past differentiates out from the present, so the future also forms as a more structured place.

Primary Dissociation This term refers to the shutting down of the functions of integration and differentiation during the traumatic process. It is passively suffered, and is an important contributor to the special characteristics of the zero process.

Secondary Dissociation (also simply Dissociation) This is a defensive process in which the ego actively takes over and uses for its own purposes the passively suffered primary dissociation of trauma. It is used, as an example, in ongoing trauma, to go somewhere else in fantasy, to be separate from the body that is being abused, etc.

Post-traumatic secondary dissociation shades into the flexible use of partial shutting down of integration and differentiation as part of the normal adaptive use of regression, which does not have to have traumatic primary dissociation as an antecedent.

Splitting of the Identity   A compound zero process defense that involves the use of the primary and secondary dissociation of the zero process combined with a special kind of counterforce defense, having properties of both repression and self/other differentiation. This unique form of counterforce is used to keep different identities, built around core zero process memories, separate.

Temporal Shifting   This is a zero process defense in which the about-to-happen, not-yet-happened nature of zero process memories is used to push the traumatic occurrence into the future (or keep it there— since in unprocessed trauma, that is where it lives in any case). The person lives at some point just before the trauma happened, and the wish to change the outcome is felt as real. Given that the zero process drive pushes traumatic memories to actualize themselves, temporal shifting gives the drive and these memories a place to live without fully intruding into the person's present life.

Universal Primal Denials   These are powerful primal denials that we all share, although the specific details of the content vary individually. These denials keep at bay full knowledge of our fragility, of our eventual death, and of the limited investment and love that those around us feel for us, and we for them. They are complex structures built of various mechanisms, such as shifting of attention, denial in fantasy, etc., and in the best case are also flexible structures, which allow reasonable acknowledgement of these realities, even as full the emotional impact is kept at bay. They are necessary protectors of our mental stability, as shown by the traumatic process that ensues when they break down too suddenly.

Zero Process   A basic form of mental functioning, to be contrasted with the secondary process and the primary process. These are the three great forms of functioning of the mind. The contents of the zero process have characteristics of both memory and immediate experience. They have the persistence over time of long-term memories, but they have the immediacy, intrusiveness, and tendency to run in one temporal direction of experience. The zero process is a product of the traumatic process—the shutting down of various levels of processing of immediate experience. Because this experience is unconstructed it does not go through the process of being laid down as more regular memories of the past but remains as a present experience, although one with special characteristics of deficient synthesis with other memories, deficient synthesis between its elements, intrusiveness through the push of the **zero process drive**, and lack of change or movement of its elements over time. The zero process memories can be processed into regular memories in the case of **bland trauma**, or can be kept from consciousness and action by repression and various **zero process defenses**, in which case they are structured as a second reality that the effected person lives within.

Zero process Defense A zero process defense is an ego (secondary process) mental action which uses some aspect of the functioning of the zero process for defensive purposes. Examples are dissociation, zero process denial, temporal shifting, and splitting of the identity.

Zero Process Denial In regular denial, there is a shifting of attention and use of other ego processes, such as suppression, minimization, and generalization, to keep full knowledge of an unpleasant reality from conscious awareness. Zero process denial adds to this the fact that, at the psychical level, the core unprocessed parts of the trauma have not yet happened. They live most of the time in the future, and so to not believe they have happened not only feels true, it is true. In this connection to placement of traumatic memories in the future, zero process denial is related to, and is usually paired with, temporal shifting.

Zero process Drive The zero process drive is the inherent push that unprocessed post-traumatic memories have towards being actualized as a lived present experience. In this continuous push, in being an independent center of motivation, and in the use of repression and other counterforce defenses to keep it from conscious experience, the zero process drive is analogous to the sexual and aggressive drives of the id. In the fact that it is tied to specific memories and is not very malleable, and in the fact that it is formed from specific experiences rather than having an inborn core, it differs from these other drives.

Zero Process Object These are commonly referred to as introjects. They are a product of trauma, and share the character of the zero process of being an immediate experience. In this they differ from regular self and object representations. They face the person as something separate from them and as an independent center of initiative, powered by the zero process drive. They do not have the malleability and changeability of other object and self representations, but rather they repeat specific scenarios of actions and reactions and comments.

References

Atkin, S. (1974). A borderline case: Ego synthesis and cognition. *International Journal of Psychoanalysis*, 55: 13–19.

Atkin, S. (1975). A borderline case: Ego synthesis and cognition: A reply to the discussion by Janice de Saussure. *International Journal of Psychoanalysis*, 56: 221–223.

Bergmann, M. S., & Jucovy, M. E. (Eds.). (1982). *Generations of the Holocaust*. New York: Basic Books.

Berlin, H. (2011). Presentation at the conference of the International Neuropsychoanalysis Society, Berlin, Germany, August 2011.

Bion, W. R. (1959). Attacks on linking. *International Journal of Psychoanalysis*, 40: 308–315.

Bion, W. R. (1962). *Learning From Experience*. New York: Basic Books.

Blum, H. P. (1974). The borderline childhood of the Wolf Man. *Journal of the American Psychoanalytic Association*, 22: 721–742.

Blum, H. P. (2013a). Introduction: the Wolf Man's Rorschach. *International Journal of Psychoanalysis*, 94: 937–944.

Blum, H. P. (2013b). Wolf Man: concluding commentary. *International Journal of Psychoanalysis*, 94: 963–966.

Botella, C. (2014). On remembering: The notion of memory without recollection. *International Journal of Psychoanalysis*, 95: 911–936.

Brenner, I. (2001). *Dissociation of Trauma: Theory, Phenomenology, and Technique.* Madison, Ct.: International Universities Press.

Brenner, I. (2004). *Psychic Trauma: Dynamics, Symptoms and Treatment*. Lanham, Mld.: Jason Aronson.

Brenner, I. (2014). *Dark Matters: Exploring the Realm of Psychic Devastation*. London: Karnac.

Breuer, J., & Freud, S. (1895). *Studies in Hysteria. S. E. 2*. London: Hogarth.

Brewin, C. R. (2003). *Post-traumatic Stress Disorder: Malady or Myth?* New Haven and London: Yale University Press.

Bromberg, N., & Small, V. V. (1983). *Hitler's Psychopathology*. New York, NY: International Universities Press.

Coates, S. W. (2016). Can babies remember trauma? Symbolic forms of re-presentation in traumatized infants. *Journal of the American Psychoanalytic Association*, 64: 751–776.

Dallaire, R. (2016). *Waiting for First Light: My Ongoing Battle With PTSD*. Toronto: Random House.

De M'Uzan, M. (2003). (Originally published in French in 1984). Slaves of Quantity. *Psychoanalytic Quarterly, 72*: 711–725.

Ferenczi, S. (1933). Confusion of tongues between adults and the child. In S. Ferenczi (1980b). *Final Contributions to the Problems and Methods of Psychoanalysis, ed. M. Balint* (pp 156–167). New York: Bruner Mazel.

Fernando, J. (2009). *The Processes of Defense: Trauma, Drives, and Reality—a New Synthesis*. Lanham, Md: Jason Aronson.

Fernando, J. (2011). Repetition and Reality: The Case of Contrast Defences. *Canadian Journal of Psychoanalysis, 19*: 279–297.

Fernando, J. (2012a). Trauma and the zero process. *Canadian Journal of Psychoanalysis, 20*: 267–290.

Fernando, J. (2012b). Trauma und der zeroprozess. *Psyche – Zeitschrift für Psychoanalyse, 66*: 1043–1073.

Fernando, J. (2013). Processes of defence: introduction to a new theory. *Canadian Journal of Psychoanalysis, 21*: 7–14.

Fonagy, P., Gergely, G., Jurist, E., & Target, M. (2002). *Affect Regulation, Mentalization, and the Development of the Self*. New York, NY: Other Press.

Fonagy, P., Luyten, P. & Strathearn, L. (2011). Borderline Personality disorder, mentalization, and the neurobiology of attachment. *Infant Mental Health Journal, 32*: 47–69.

Frank, A. (1969). The unrememberable and the unforgettable: passive primal repression. *Psychoanalytic Study of the Child, 24*: 48–77.

Freud, A. (1936). *The Ego and the Mechanisms of Defense*. New York: International Universities Press.

Freud, S. (1900). *The Interpretation of Dreams. S. E. 4–5*. London: Hogarth.

Freud, S. (1905). Three essays on the theory of sexuality. *S. E. 7*: 123–245. London: Hogarth.

Freud, S. (1910). The Psycho-Analytic View of Psychogenic Disturbance of Vision. *S.E. 9*: 209–221. London: Hogarth.

Freud, S. (1912). The dynamics of transference. *S. E. 12*: 97–108. London: Hogarth.

Freud, S. (1914). On the History of the Psycho-Analytic Movement. *S. E. 14*: 1–66. London: Hogarth.

Freud, S. (1915). Observations on transference love (further recommendations on the technique of psychoanalysis III). *S. E 12*: 157–171. London: Hogarth.

Freud, S. (1917 [1915]). Mourning and melancholia. *S. E. 14*: 237–258. London: Hogarth.

Freud, S. (1918). From the history of an infantile neurosis. *S. E., 17*: 1–123.

Freud, S. (1920). *Beyond the Pleasure Principle. S. E., 18*: 1–64. London: Hogarth.

Freud, S. (1921). *Group Psychology and the Analysis of the Ego. S. E. 18*: 65–143. London: Hogarth.

Freud, S. (1923). *The Ego and the Id. S.E. 19*: 1–66. London: Hogarth.

Freud, S. (1925). A note upon the 'mystic writing-pad'. *S. E. 19*: 225–232. London: Hogarth.

Freud, S. (1926). Inhibitions, symptoms and anxiety. *S. E., 20*: 75–175.

Freud, S. (1937). Constructions in analysis. *S. E., 23*: 255–269.

Freud, S. (1940). Splitting of the ego in the process of defense. *S. E. 23*: 271–278. London: Hogarth.

Furst, S. S. (1978). The stimulus barrier and the pathogenicity of trauma. *International Journal of Psychoanalysis, 59*: 345–352.

Gaensbauer, T. J. (1994). Therapeutic work with a traumatized toddler. *Psychoanalytic Study of the Child, 49*: 412–433.

Gaensbauer, T. J. (1995). Trauma in the preverbal period: symptoms, memories, and developmental impact. *Psychoanalytic Study of the Child, 50*: 122–149.

Gaensbauer, T. J., & Jordan, L. (2009). Psychoanalytic perspectives on early trauma: interviews with thirty analysts who treated an adult victim of a circumscribed trauma in early childhood. *Journal of the American Psychoanalytic Association, 57*: 947–977.

Gill, M. M., & Brenman, M. (1961). *Hypnosis and Related States: Psychoanalytic Studies in Regression*. New York: International Universities Press.

Greenacre, P. (1967). The influence of infantile trauma on genetic patterns. In S. S. Furst (Ed.), *Psychic Trauma*. (pp. 108–153). New York: Basic Books.

Grubrich-Simitis, I. (2010). Reality testing in place of interpretation: a phase in psychoanalytic work with descendants of holocaust survivors. *Psychoanalytic Quarterly, 79*: 37–69.

Hartmann, H. (1939). *Ego Psychology and the Problem of Adaptation*. Translated by D. Rappaport (1958 edition). New York: International Universities Press.

Hartmann, H. (1948). Comments on the psychoanalytic theory of the instinctual drives. *Psychoanalytic Quarterly, 17*: 368–388.

Hartmann, H. (1950). Comments on the psychoanalytic theory of the ego. *Psychoanalytic Study of the Child, 5*: 74–96.

Hartmann, H. (1953). Contributions to the metapsychology of schizophrenia. *Psychoanalytic Study of the Child, 8*: 177–198.

Hartmann, H. (1955). Notes on the Theory of Sublimation. *Psychoanalytic Study of the Child, 10*: 9–29.

Hartmann, H., Kris, E., & Loewenstein, R. M. (1946). Comments on the Formation of Psychic Structure. *Psychoanalytic Study of the Child, 2*: 11–38.

Hartmann, H. Kris, E., & Loewenstein, R. M. (1949). Notes on the Theory of Aggression. *Psychoanalytic Study of the Child, 3*: 9–36.

Hock, U. (2014). Plea for the unity of the Freudian theory of memory. *International Journal of Psychoanalysis, 95*: 937–950.

Howell, E. (2005). *The Dissociative Mind*. New York: Routledge.

Hurvich, M. (2003). The place of annihilation anxieties in psychoanalytic theory. *Journal of the American Psychoanalytic Association, 51*: 579–616.

Jacobson, E. (1957). Denial and repression. *Journal of the American Psychoanalytic Association, 5*: 61–92.

Jacobson, E. (1964). *The Self and the Object World*. New York: International Universities Press.

Janet, P. (1920). *The Major Symptoms of Hysteria (2nd ed)*. New York, NY: The MacMillan Company.

Janet (1932). Les croyances et les hallucinations. *Revue Philosophique, 113*: 278–331.

Kernberg, O. (1967). Borderline Personality Organization. *Journal of the American Psychoanalytic Association, 15*: 641–685.

Kernberg, O. (1975). *Borderline Conditions and Pathological Narcissism*. New York, NY: Jason Aronson.

Kernberg, O. F. (2019). Therapeutic implications of transference structures in various personality pathologies. *Journal of the American Psychoanalytic Association, 67*: 951–986.

Kestenberg, J. S. (1980). Psychoanalyses of children of survivors from the holocaust: case presentations and assessment. *Journal of the American Psychoanalytic Association, 28*: 775–804.

Kestenberg, J. S. (1993). What a Psychoanalyst Learned from the Holocaust and Genocide. *International Journal of Psychoanalysis, 74*: 1117–1129.

Klein, M. (1945). The Oedipus Complex in the Light of Early Anxieties. *International Journal of Psychoanalysis, 26*: 11–33.

Klein, M. (1946). Notes on some schizoid mechanisms. *International Journal of Psychoanalysis, 27*: 99–110.

Klein, M. (1958). On the Development of Mental Functioning. *International Journal of Psychoanalysis, 39*: 84–90.

Kluft, R. P. (Ed). (1985a). *Childhood Antecedents of Multiple Personality*. DC: American Psychiatric Press.

Kluft, R. P. (1985b). Childhood multiple personality disorder: predictors, clinical findings, and treatment results. In R. P. Kluft (Ed.), (1985). *Childhood Antecedents of Multiple Personality* (pp. 167–196). DC: American Psychiatric Press.

Kluft, R. P. (1997). On the treatment of traumatic memories of DID patients: Always? Never? Sometimes? Now? Later? *Dissociation 10*(2): 80–90.

Kluft, R. P. (2000). The psychoanalytic psychotherapy of dissociative identity disorder in the context of trauma therapy. *Psychoanalytic Inquiry 20*: 259–286.

Kluft, R. P. (2013). *Shelter from the Storm: Processing the memories of DID/DDNOS Patients with the Fractionated Abreaction Technique*. North Charleston, S.C: Create Space Independent Publishing Platform.

Koch, E. (2012). The Hampstead clinic at Work. Discussions in the diagnostic profile research group. *Psychoanalytic Study of the Child, 66*: 281–315.

Kris, E. (1950). On preconscious mental processes. *Psychoanalytic Quarterly, 19*: 540–560.

Kris, E. (1955). Neutralization and Sublimation—Observations on Young Children. *Psychoanalytic Study of the Child, 10*: 30–46.

Kris, E. (1956a). On some vicissitudes of insight in psychoanalysis. *International Journal of Psychoanalysis, 37*: 445–455.

Kris, E. (1956b). The recovery of childhood memories in psychoanalysis. *Psychoanalytic Study of the Child, 11*: 54–88.

Levine, H. B., Reed, G. S., & Scarfone, D. (Eds.). (2013). *Unrepresented States and the Construction of Meaning: Clinical and Theoretical Contributions*. London: Karnac.

Lipin, T. (1963). The repetition compulsion and the "maturational" drive-representatives. *International Journal of Psycho-Analysis, 44*: 389–406.

Loewenstein, R. J. (1993). Dissociation, Development, and the Psychobiology of Trauma. *Journal of the American Academy of Psychoanalysis, 21*: 581–603.

Loewenstein, R. J., & Ross, D. R. (1992). multiple personality and psychoanalysis: an introduction. *Psychoanalytic Inquiry, 12*: 3–48.

Mahler, M. S. (1971). A study of the separation-Individuation process—and its possible application to borderline phenomena in the psychoanalytic situation. *Psychoanalytic Study of the Child*, 26: 403–424.

Mahler, M. S., Pine, F., & Bergman, A. (1975). *The Psychological Birth of the Human Infant*. U.S.A: Basic Books.

Maldonado, J. R., & Spiegel, D. (1998). Trauma, dissociation, and hypnotizability. In Bremner, J. D. & Marmar, C. R. (Ed). (1998). *Trauma, Memory, and Dissociation* (pp. 57–106). Washington, D. C.: American Psychiatric Press.

Marty, P. (1968). A Major Process of Somatization: The Progressive Disorganization. *International Journal of Psychoanalysis*, 49: 246–249.

Matthis, I., & Deutsch, J. (2005). International society of Neuro-psychoanalysis, Toronto group. *Neuro-Psychoanalysis*, 7: 228–229.

Micale, M. S. & Lerner, P. (eds). (2001). *Traumatic Pasts: History, Psychiatry and Trauma in the Modern Age, 1870–1930*. New York: Cambridge University Press.

Moskowitz, A., Heim, G., Saillot, I., & Beavan, V. (2019). Pierre Janet on hallucinations, paranoia, and schizophrenia. In Craparo, G., Ortu, F. and van der Hart, O. (eds.) (2019), *Rediscovering Pierre Janet: Trauma, Dissociation, and a new Context for Psychoanalysis* (pp. 130–142). New York, NY: Routledge.

Niederland, W. G. (1965). The role of the ego in the recovery of early memories. *Psychoanalytic Quarterly*, 34: 564–571.

Niederland, W. G. (1981). The survivor syndrome: further observations and dimensions. *Journal of the American Psychoanalytic Association*, 29: 413–425.

Novick, J., & Novick, K. K. (1996). *Fearful Symmetry: The Development and Treatment of Sadomasochism*. Northvale, NJ: Jason Aronson.

Ogden, P., Minton, K., & Pain, C. (2006). *Trauma and the Body: A Sensorimotor Approach to Psychotherapy*. New York and London: Norton.

Phillips, S. H. (1991). Trauma and war: a fragment of an analysis with a Vietnam veteran. *Psychoanalytic Study of the Child 46*, 147–180.

Putnam, F. W. (1989). *Diagnosis and Treatment of Multiple Personality Disorder*. New York: Guilford.

Riley, R. L., & Mead, J. (1988). The development of symptoms of multiple personality disorder in a child of three. *Dissociation 1*: 41–46.

Rousillon, R. (2011). *Primitive Agony and Symbolization*. London: Karnac Books.

Sandberg, L. S., & Tortora, S. (2019). Thinking (and moving) outside of the box: psychoanalytic treatment and dance/movement therapy. *Psychoanalytic Quarterly*, 88: 839–865.

Scarfone, D. (2006). A Matter of Time: Actual Time and the Production of the Past. *Psychoanalytic Quarterly*, 75: 807–834.

Scarfone, D. (2014). The work of remembering and the revival of the psychoanalytic method. *International Journal of Psychoanalysis*, 95: 965–972.

Scarfone, D. (2015). *The Unpast: The Actual Unconscious*. New York: The Unconscious in Translation.

Schacter, D. L. (1996). *Searching for Memory*. New York: Basic Books.

Schacter, D. L. (2001). *The Seven Sins of Memory: How the Mind Forgets and Remembers*. New York: Houghton Mifflin.

Schreiber, F. R. (1973). *Sybil*. New York, New York: Warner Books.

Shengold, L. (1988). *Halo in the Sky: Observations on Anality and Defense*. New Haven: Yale University Press.

Shengold, L. (1989). *Soul Murder: The Effects of Childhood Abuse and Deprivation*. New York: Fawcett.

Shevrin, H. (2002). A psychoanalytic view of memory in the light of recent cognitive and neuroscience research. *Neuropsychoanalysis, 4*: 131–139.

Sodré, I. (2019) Through the looking glass: on trauma and unreality. *International Journal of Psycho-Analysis, 100*: 1171–1183.

Stern, A. (1938). Psychoanalytic Investigation of and Therapy in the Border Line Group of Neuroses. *Psychoanalytic Quarterly, 7*: 467–489.

Stern, A. (1945). Psychoanalytic Therapy in the Borderline Neuroses. *Psychoanalytic Quarterly, 14*: 190–198.

Terr, L. (1995). *Unchained Memories: True Stories of Traumatic Memories Lost and Found*. New York: Basic Books.

Terr, L. C. (2013). What becomes of infantile traumatic memories?: an adult "wild child" is asked to remember. *Psychoanalytic Study of the Child, 67*: 197–214.

Van der Hart, O., & Friedman, B. (2019). A reader's guide to Pierre Janet: a neglected intellectual heritage. In Craparo, G., Ortu, F. & van der Hart, O. (eds.) (2019), *Rediscovering Pierre Janet: Trauma, Dissociation, and a new Context for Psychoanalysis* (pp. 4–27). New York, NY: Routledge.

Van Der Kolk, B. (2014). *The Body Keeps Score: Brain, Mind, and Body in the Healing of Trauma*. N.Y., New York: Penguin.

Van Der Kolk, B., & Van Der Hart, O. (1995). The intrusive past: the flexibility of memory and the engraving of trauma. In C. Caruth (Ed.), *Trauma: Explorations in Memory* (pp. 158–182). Baltimore: Johns Hopkins University Press.

Van Der Kolk, B., Van der Hart, O., & Marmar, C. R. (1996). Dissociation and information processing in post-traumatic stress disorder. In B. Van der Kolk, A. C. McFarlane, & L. Weissreth (Eds.), *Traumatic Stress: The Effects of Overwhelming Experience on Mind, Body and Society* (pp. 303–327). New York: Guilford.

Volkan, V. D. (2014). *Psychoanalysis, International Relations, and Diplomacy: A Sourcebook on Large-Group Psychology*. London: Karnac.

Volkan, V. D. (2015). *A Nazi Legacy: Depositing, Transgenerational Transmission, Dissociation, and Remembering Through Action*. London: Karnac.

Winnicott, D. W. (1974). Fear of Breakdown. *International Review of Psychoanalysis, 1*: 103–107.

Index